Perspectives on Vision

Selected papers from the
Kraskin Invitational
Skeffington Symposium
on Vision
1984 to 1989

Compiled by Paul A. Harris, O.D.

Optometric Extension Program Foundation

Copyright © 2003
Optometric Extension Program Foundation, Inc.

Printed in the United States

Published by the Optometric Extension Program
1921 E. Carnegie Ave., Suite 3-L
Santa Ana, CA 92705-5510

Managing editor: Sally Marshall Corngold
Cover design: Kathleen Patterson

Library of Congress Cataloging-in-Publication Data pending
ISBN 0-943599-47-4

****

Optometry is the health care profession specifically licensed by state law to prescribe lenses, optical devices and procedures to improve human vision. Optometry has advanced vision therapy as a unique treatment modality for the development and remediation of the visual process. Effective vision therapy requires extensive understanding of:
the effects of lenses (including prisms, filters and occluders)
the variety of responses to the changes produced by lenses
the various physiological aspects of the visual process
the pervasive nature of the visual process in human behavior

As a consequence, effective vision therapy requires the supervision, direction and active involvement of the optometrist.

****

Table of Contents

Introduction..i

1984

1. Notes to be Read Before the First Examination 1
   Bruce Wolff, OD
2. Beyond Harmon: Aspects of a Psycho-Behavioral Philosophy..........6
   Elliott Forrest, OD
3. Zen and the Art of Vision Maintenance............................14
   Barry Millis, OD

1985

4. Involuntary Focus and Convergence at the Resting State 19
   Ronald Shane, OD

1986

5. Visual Imagery and the Plateau Spiral in Myopia Control 31
   Elliott Forrest, OD
6. The Use of Base-Down Prism in the Treatment of the
   Cerebral Palsied Patient...36
   Wendy Garson, OD
7. Eye Movements, Information Theory, and the Rule of Language....42
   Ronald Berger, OD

1987

8. Observations on Characteristics of Distance Blur 52
   Gregory Kitchener, OD
9. The Gesellian contributions and Their Impact Upon our
   Optometric Heritage 55
   G.N. Getman, OD

1988

10. What is 'The Core Philosophy?' 66
    G.N. Getman, OD
11. Nearpoint Lens Prescriptions: Clinical Methods for Comparing
    and Evaluating Selected Dynamic Retinoscopy Techniques 77
    Harold Haynes, OD
12. The Impact of Visual Training on Intelligence 106
    Martin Kane, OD

1989

13. The Interplay Between Change and Restraint 114
    Barry Millis, OD
14. The Baltimore Myopia Control Project –
    A Major Turning Point 119
    G.N. Getman, OD

Introduction

Paul A. Harris, O.D., Editor

Robert A. Kraskin, O.D., was fond of quoting, "The past is prologue to the future."[1] With a better knowledge of the past, which established the foundation upon which our clinical discipline develops, each of us is better prepared to meet what the future holds. A parallel idea is that, often, new discoveries are not new at all. There are notions, ideas, theories, or concepts that re-emerge in the collective consciousness from time to time for inspection. Often it seems that a new thought, idea, or theory emerges, but in reality it is a new packaging for something that has been around for a long time.

In a videotape recorded during a seminar by the late Bruce Wolff, O.D., in 1985, he stopped during his presentation and surveyed the group about their exposure to specific people and knowledge of particular pieces of information. The majority had never heard A.M. Skeffington or Darell Boyd Harmon and had never seen the Harmon videos. Bruce then commented that one of the most difficult things for speakers to keep in mind is how much experience and knowledge is in their own minds which they then take for granted co-exists in the minds of the audience.

For all of these reasons this volume presents selected papers from what is now named the Kraskin Invitational Skeffington Symposium on Vision (KISS). Those familiar with these papers from 15-20 years ago have the opportunity to experience them from the new perspective of their continued growth and development. This volume covers the time period of 1984 to 1989.

NOTE: Because these are transcripts of oral presentations, reference citations are not formally done. This is not a refereed publication.

---

[1] *The National Archives and Records Administration, 8601 Adelphi Rd., College Park, MD 20740-6001 www.archives.gov. The inscription "The Past is Prologue" appears on a statue outside of the NARA building in Washington, DC, on Pennsylvania Avenue. The female statue, representing the Future, is inscribed with a line inspired by Shakespeare's play The Tempest (Act 2, Scene 1, line 261): "What is Past is Prologue."*

The Nature of the Meeting

The KISS meeting, affectionately called "The Skeffington" for short, has been held in the Washington, D.C., area each January for nearly 50 years. It is a meeting designed for 20 people, which generally has many times that. The meeting is strictly for optometrists and includes two types of registrants: presenters and non-presenters. Presenters submit a paper ahead of time and the moderator and chairman decide the schedule of presentations, but the presenters have no more than a few moments notice when it is their turn.

A moderated discussion follows the presentation of the paper. Some are short, conceptual papers presented for the purpose of triggering dialogue on a subject. In these instances the "meat" of the paper is in the discussion. Since no transcripts of the dialogues exist, papers of this type were not selected for this volume.

Often presenters would work the entire year preparing their paper for the next meeting. This is reflected in the very high quality of many of the papers. KISS afforded forward thinkers a forum to try out a new idea or a new insight and to get critical feedback from colleagues in an open, no-holds-barred environment that fostered collegial exchange.

Paper Selection

The papers selected for inclusion in this volume are those that either (1) presented new ideas that foreshadowed future developments, (2) presented new clinical procedures or thinking that have become part of the standard repertoire of behavioral vision care, (3) presented the particulars and/or history of a watershed event in our heritage or (4) presented a body of work that merits critical review in the light of new knowledge.

Selecting just 14 papers for this anthology was a difficult task. Complete transcripts of all the papers for each year are available from the Optometric Extension Program Foundation for those who are interested.[2] The following is a brief description of each of the papers in this limited selection. These are arranged in chronological order.

---

[2] *Croissant Transcripts. Optometric Extension Program Foundation, 1921 E. Carnegie Ave., Ste. 3-L, Santa Ana, CA 92705, (949) 250-8070.*

The Papers

1984

Notes to be Read Before the First Examination
Bruce Wolff, O.D.

Bruce Wolff, O.D, began this brief paper. John Streff, O.D., and Sr. Barbara Jinks, O.P., M.A., contributed to the final product. It was developed during their work together at the Skeffington Alexander National Optometric Education Learning Center (s.a. NOEL Center) in Lancaster, Ohio. Bruce Wolff, who A.M. Skeffington entrusted with his personal vision care, influenced the development of many in the profession. This he did primarily as a mentor, teacher, and clinician (sometimes antagonist) and not primarily through the written word. Many of us struggle with how to use language to communicate to the public what we do. It is interesting to see how these three set the stage for the examination with this short paper given to patients prior to coming to the office.

Beyond Harmon: Aspects of a Psycho-Behavioral Philosophy
Elliott Forrest, O.D.

In this paper Dr. Forrest shares many of the ideas that triggered the development of his Psycho-Behavioral philosophy of vision care. To help understand his change in perspective he begins by deciphering some of the groundbreaking work of Darrell Boyd Harmon on the intertwined relationships of posture and vision. Forrest shows us that Harmon's way of looking at these relationships dealt primarily with the forces and actions interacting on the physical level. This is analogous to the early work of Hans Selye and Walter B. Cannon who described stresses acting on the organism to produce a stress effect. These interactions were seen to occur in the physical world in much the same manner as the forces Harmon saw acting on the individual.

Dr. Forrest suggests that persons and their minds are the actual site of the interaction between the postural demands on persons and their corporeal selves. This was similar to the way modern stress theory added modulator functions such as *attitude, appraisal, intensity,* etc., to the stress equations. This drastically altered the site at which stressors acted or were modified. This paper will help readers of Dr. Forrest's *Stress and Vision*[3] understand the early beginnings of his insights.

---

[3] *Forrest E. Stress and Vision. Optometric Extension Program Foundation, 1921 E. Carnegie Ave., Ste. 3-L, Santa Ana, CA 92705, (949) 250-8070.*

Zen and the Art of Vision Maintenance
Barry Millis, O.D.
This intriguing paper presents important and critical information for every optometrist who provides any behavioral vision care services and attempts to communicate with the rest of the human race about what those services are. Dr. Millis illuminates what many take for granted at one level and, at another level, lose sight of regularly. Many in the public perceive behavioral aspects of vision care as not much different than any other eye/vision care services. He states, "Behavioral optometry is like the shift from Newton's physics to Einstein's physics – there is a fundamental change in perspective." His paper puts forward concepts for us to think about and chew on. These should remain front and center in our minds from that point forward when talking with other people about *vision*.

1985

Involuntary Focus and Convergence at the Resting State
Ronald Shane, O.D.
With this paper Dr. Shane brings attention to concepts that upset many of the embedded ideas about the mechanism of accommodation. He introduces data about the dark focus, negative accommodation, the Mandelbaum effect and many other insights into accommodation. He also includes simple practical clinical procedures to explore the dark focus and its affect on a person's use of accommodation in a wide range of conditions to derive meaning and direct action.

1986

Visual Imagery and the Plateau Spiral in Myopia Control
Elliott Forrest, O.D.
This short paper presents four activities using the Plateau spiral with a patient working on myopia control. Visual imagery[4] was a topic near and dear to Dr. Forrest. He gives the history of the use of the Plateau spiral and innovations using visual imagery. Mastery of the technique allows a person to "enlarge" or "bring closer" something that they couldn't otherwise see clearly enough to discern.

---

[4] *Forrest E. Visual Imagery. Optometric Extension Program Foundation, 1921 E. Carnegie Ave., Ste. 3-L, Santa Ana, CA 92705, (949) 250-8070.*

The Use of Base Down Prism in the Treatment of the Cerebral Palsied Patient
Wendy Garson, O.D.
Dr. Garson presents information on her use of prisms to help patients with cerebral palsy. The prisms alter the muscle tone in their bodies when there is a gross imbalance between extension and flexion. Here the prisms are not used directly to improve the clarity of sight or to compensate for a specific visual spatial misalignment. Instead, the prisms are used to set the stage for the person to achieve a better balance within their body so that dynamic muscle tension can be reduced. The result is better and smoother movements and a reduction of spasticity.

Eye Movements, Information Theory and the Rule of Language
Ronald Berger, O.D.
This is the first paper given by Dr. Berger on language and vision, a topic of great interest for him. Various devices are used to record and analyze eye movements while reading text. His premise is that to understand how a person parses text (the pattern of fixations and regression over time), we should better understand how information is stored in language. He recounts the groundbreaking work done by Claude Shannon and Norbert Wiener. Their work in the fields of electronic communications and cryptology exposed the high degree of redundancy built into languages. Readers may use a simpler pattern of eye movements when reading a passage that conforms to their current language patterns than when reading a passage that follows a different pattern of language rules. These relationships are fundamental to understanding eye movement patterns for deriving meaning when dealing with language symbols. Dr. Berger has continued to develop this understanding.

1987

Observations on Characteristics of Distance Blur
Gregory Kitchener, O.D.
In this paper Dr. Kitchener uses the paper by Dr. Forrest on the Plateau spiral as a jumping off point. He takes the thread begun by Dr. Forrest and presents a clinical probe that he uses to yield clinical insights into many of the facets of *vision* proposed by Dr. Forrest. He observes that, under some conditions, patients report apparent paradoxes that are

based in the mind of the patient. These reflect how the patient has organized the representation of reality in the mind's eye.

The Gesellian Contributions and Their Impact Upon our Optometric Heritage
G.N. Getman, O.D.

In this paper, presented at the Sunday brunch, Dr. Getman describes how a simple chance changed the face of our profession. Getman was scheduled to leave Baltimore, MD, after his two weeks of clinical service on the Baltimore Myopia Project. His departure was delayed as all trains were reserved for troop movements that day. This happened to be the day that Arnold Gesell, M.D., came to visit the study. The two became acquainted as they spent most of the day together outside the clinic. Dr. Getman calls the impact of the Gesellian contributions one of the five most important events to shape optometry. Who better to tell it than the optometrist who spent the most time working alongside Dr. Gesell?

1988

What is "The Core Philosophy?"
G.N. Getman, O.D.

In this paper Dr. Getman provides his perspective on language used to describe what we do. As a vehicle to elaborate what Behavioral Optometry is to him, he uses six statements that he labels "dogmas." An example is, "Vision is the dominant process in human behavior," attributed to Arnold Gesell, M.D. Dr. Getman proposes rephrasing this, as well as the other frequently repeated statements of dogma. In the process of working through these statements Dr. Getman moves through these basic tenets of behavioral vision care giving each fuller meaning. These changes set the stage for better understanding and acceptance of these foundational concepts by others outside the profession.

Nearpoint Lens Prescriptions: Clinical Methods for Comparing and Evaluating Selected Dynamic Retinoscopy Techniques
Harold Haynes, O.D.

As a researcher and teacher, Dr. Harold Haynes developed Monocular Estimation Method (MEM) retinoscopy as a clinical tool used by many. The latter part of the 20th century saw a great deal of interest in exploiting retinoscopic observations. Several different procedures or methods for gaining insight into human behavior from observations of the light reflected from a retinoscope were developed during this period. Each had their proponents and dialogue about which was the best or the "right" one abounded. The contributions of Robert Kraskin, Darrel Boyd Harmon, Harold Haynes, Jerry Getman, Richard Apell, and John Streff are influential in our clinical understanding of the retinoscope. In this paper Dr. Haynes attempts to unify or equate four of the most well-known retinoscopy techniques. Dr. Haynes' meticulous work and presentations always triggered lively dialogue. This paper was no exception.

The Impact of Visual Training on Intelligence
Martin Kane, O.D.
Traditionally, the KISS officially started on Saturday afternoon with a paper by Dr. Martin Kane. This paper systematically evaluates the seven areas of intelligence proposed by Howard Gardner's theory of multiple intelligences. Dr. Kane demonstrates vision training's potential to affect the development of and use of these intelligences. Understanding this paper can help when communicating with educators and psychologists. In *How to Develop Your Child's Intelligence,*[5] Dr. Jerry Getman asserted that as we provide children with necessary, meaningful experiences in life they develop not only visual abilities, but also intelligence. Dr. Harry Wachs asserts that people create intelligence as they develop and learn. Dr. Kane provides insight into an even broader use of these concepts.

1989

The Interplay Between Change and Restraint
Barry Millis, O.D.
In this paper Dr. Millis tackles head on the challenge of answering the question, "Is it nature or is it nurture?" *Of Mind and Nature – A Necessary Unity*[6] by Gregory Bateson and Elliott Forrest's *Stress and Vision* are used to address this frequently asked question. A full understanding of this paper can sharpen the reader's ability to answer this type of question whenever and wherever it crops up.

---

[5] *Getman G. How to Develop Your Child's Intelligence. Optometric Extension Program Foundation, 1921 E. Carnegie Ave., Ste. 3-L, Santa Ana, CA 92705, (949) 250-8070.*
[6] *Bateson G. Of Mind and Nature – A Necessary Unity. Bantam Books 1979*

The Baltimore Myopia Control Project – A Major Turning Point
G.N. Getman, O.D.
In this final selection, Dr. Getman discusses another of the five most important events in the history of our profession. This project took place near the end of World War II, beginning in the fall of 1944 and finishing early in 1945. Others have reported on the specific data from this research. Dr. Getman details six lessons optometry learned that became fundamental to establishing behavioral aspects of vision care. Dr. Getman marks this study as, "The turning point of the profession from its infancy to childhood." Many take for granted the lessons learned during the execution of the study.

Acknowledgments

Drs. Robert A. Kraskin and Paul Lewis and their families deserve many thanks for the success of this meeting. During these years, 1984-1989, Bob Kraskin chaired each meeting and Paul Lewis served as moderator. Under their guidance the meeting maintained an intensity and collegiality that is hard to match in any other setting. The two sat together at the front of the room deciding the order of presentations. When appropriate they would interject comments to provide an historical perspective or insights from other professions.

Hopefully these selections provide the reader with some feeling of what it was like to actually attend the meeting. Maybe the reader can also experience some of the "ah-ha's" and reorganization of concepts that affected many of the meetings' participants.

Notes to be Read Before the First Examination

Bruce Wolff, O.D.
Cincinnati, OH

About Vision

The purpose of this pamphlet is to provide information that will make it easier for you to more quickly understand the results of the examination and any treatment that may be prescribed. While it is intended primarily for those who are making their first visit, others may find it equally useful.

It may be of interest to you to know sources of referral and reasons for coming other than your own. Referral sources vary: those in education, the medical community, books and other materials written for the general public, and people who either have been patients or know patients. The reasons also can be quite varied: a formal vision screening of some kind, inadequate academic performance problems, a last resort for undefined and so far insoluble problems, and rehabilitation (and occasionally enhancement) of visual abilities that are essential to meet particular visual eligibility requirements.

Whatever the source of referral or the particular reason for coming, two questions asked are outstanding in the frequency of their occurrence:

1. Is something really wrong?
2. Can anything be done about it?

Close behind in order of frequency are:

3. What do you do in an examination?
4. What does vision have to do with my kind of problems?

Here are the easiest answers to the questions as they are stated above. Questions one and two are taken together for they are interrelated. It is remotely possible that an abnormal individual will be found in which there is little or no potential for any form of successful treatment. This category is extremely rare. Too often in the process of diagnosing and labeling, an abnormal can be "created," particularly by those unfamiliar with current levels of understanding of vision and the visual processes. The vast majority are normal persons in difficulty and can be helped to varying degrees depending upon: (1) The evidence of the available potential, (2) the embeddedness of substitute and compensating behaviors, (3) the value of different and better performance to the individual and those immediately involved, (4) and reasonable adherence to and support of the program prescribed.

The assessment made from the examination data determines what must be done and can be done.

Now question three. The examination consists of these five parts:

1. The interview

Here we ask for your reasons for coming and gather pertinent background information.

2. Screening for pathology

From this we may find pathology that has not been previously recognized (that is, not given in the interview) and is readily observable in a visual examination. For example, the obvious are cataracts and glaucoma; less obvious are indications of diabetes or hypertension. You will be informed of anything found needing referral.

3. Examining the characteristics of <u>visual space</u> and the functions of <u>centering, identification</u> and <u>binocularity</u> within it.

<u>Visual Space</u> is that space shared by those in the same place, at the same time. It involves what we see now; and what we have seen (visual memory), and what we can visualize in the future. It is formed by the combination of light from the external world and the particular environments within which one developed and learned to use.

<u>Centering</u> – the equivalent of looking to "where" in the visual space. It is the ability to direct the visual system to a volume of visual space within which identification is taking place.

<u>Identification</u> – the visual process of seeing "what" is within the visual space. It is the continuous recognition and utilization of form and the relationship of forms.

Binocularity – the process that develops from centering and identification within the visual space. It resolves similarities and differences simultaneously into unique percepts.

The bits of information that can be identified in one glance are enormous and points to one of the reasons vision is dominant.

Not exactly easy to understand, you say. True, but hang in there, it will begin to clear later. If this is your first encounter with these ideas, it is certain that you will have to think about it awhile and perhaps re-read some parts. And, you will have the opportunity to discuss and ask questions about any part of this pamphlet after the examination.

4. Integrations of the visual with the body postural and movement mechanisms, speech-auditory-language systems and those activities generally regarded as perceptual.

In the previous section, we indicated that visual space is developed through experiences. This means "doing and acting" for seeing is a motor system as well as sensory. We see to act not just to see. Thus, in this examination, we observe the visual-motor, visual-verbal, visual-auditory, and visual-perceptual and consider the contribution of vision to each of these systems, and the quality of their interaction.

5. Assessment and recommendations.

At this time the examination data is presented, translated, and compared from in-office performance on the test battery to performance characteristics in the every day world. These two must be in agreement. One consequence at this point may be a change in the order of problems to be treated due to a new awareness of all that is involved. Treatment alternatives are presented and the consequences of each discussed. Any necessary referrals to other disciplines will be made at this time. All of the results of the examination are recorded and some but not all of the original test data are retained. Those who are responsible for deciding what course of action is to be taken or who are interested in the assessment and recommendations are expected to be present and to have read this pamphlet. Brief summaries for other professionals will be given by telephone.

You may have recognized that the brief description of the examination given above hints at the answer to question four and how vision extends itself into many, many activities.

Vision is an enormously complex information process that dominates human behavior. It is so much a part of us that it is difficult to stand back and look at it. We reveal how much vision is a part of us by correctly using expressions such as "He is a man of vision," "It looks hot," "Let me see if I can remember," "He failed to foresee." Do you "see" the point? Vision is all of these: sight, hindsight, foresight and insight.

When attention is turned to and focused on the term "vision" it is almost invariably associated with and equated to "visual acuity." The most famous measure of average acuity is the Snellen fraction 20/20. But visual acuity is only a part of the total visual process. There is a profound difference between the many functions of vision and the single function of visual acuity. The understanding of those functions helps clarify how vision can be involved in so many human activities and problems.

The publication in 1949 of *Vision: Its Development in Infant and Child* by Arnold Gesell was a major contribution to the available literature that documented the elaborate nature and importance of vision. More publications have become available for the general public since then, some of which are listed in the bibliography at the end of this paper, as well as earlier ones. These references are for those who are interested in more detailed and varied information than can be contained in this brief pamphlet.

Prepared by the Executive Staff of the S.A. NOEL center, a non-profit institution for teaching and research in vision for education and optometry.

Bruce Wolff, OD
Sr. Barbara A. Jinks, O.P., M.A.
John W. Streff, OD

Bibliography
Bates WH. The Cure of Imperfect Sight by Treatment Without Glasses. New York:Central Fixation, 1920.
Huxley A. The Art of Seeing. New York:Harper, 1942.

Corbett MD. Help Yourself to Better Sight. New York:Prentice-Hall, 1949.

Gesell A. Gesell A, Ilg FL, Bullis GE. Vision – Its Development in Infant and Child. Santa Ana, CA:Optometric Extension Program Foundation, 1998. Originally published by Harper and Row, Darien, CT, 1949.

Kepes G. Language of Vision. Chicago:Paul Theobald, 1951.

Arnheim R. Visual Thinking. Berkeley and Los Angeles:University of California Press, 1969.

Ames LB, Gillespie C, Streff JW. Stop School Failure. New York:Harper & Row, 1972.

Kavner R, Dunsky L. Total Vision. New York:A.& W, 1978.

Hoopes A, Hoopes T. Eye Power. New York: Alfred A. Knopf, 1979.

Lyons EB. How to Use Your Power of Visualization. Willits, CA:Golden Rule Printing, 1980.

Forrest EB. Visual Imagery: An Optometric Approach. Santa Ana, CA: Optometric Extension Program Foundation, Inc., 1981.

Beyond Harmon: Aspects of a Personal Psycho-Behavioral Philosophy

Elliott B. Forrest, O.D., FAAO
New York, NY

Darell Boyd Harmon and the Role Of Posture

It is interesting how people get where they are in their profession. A.M. Skeffington, for example, started out by studying for the ministry. Piaget began as a biologist, became an epistemologist and wound up as one of the founders of what is now called cognitive psychology. Darell Boyd Harmon, on the other hand, got a Ph.D. at a time when graduate schools stressed a synthesis of knowledge rather than specialization. Not feeling that he was an expert in anything, he described himself as a consulting educationist simply because, as he put it, the term was meaningless. As an "educationist" he was involved with pediatrics, kinesiology, architecture, lighting, engineering, pedagogy, human performance and vision. Harmon, in fact, claimed that it was he who first got Arnold Gesell of the Yale Institute of Child Development interested in vision and visual development. Though Harmon was not an optometrist, his scope of knowledge was such that it left a strong imprint on behavioral optometry.

Harmon[1] stressed that vision was more than a high-order skill, that it was integrally related to so-called lower-order gravitational mechanisms. He conceived the organism to be constructed of three basic referential coordinate systems: the torso with its righting and counterbalancing reflexes; the head with its gravitationally-oriented vestibular mechanisms; and the visual system with the unified action of the two foveas (or a single fovea in the case of a monocular individual) acting as, what Henry Gossfeld called, a space center or a spatial referential benchmark.[2] Harmon also conceived of the neck as being the transducer mechanism between the actions of the trunk and the actions of the head and visual system.

Each of these individual coordinate systems, to Harmon, establishes its own functional invariant axis. Operationally, these separate invariants are integrated to form a composite organismic invariant axis around the "y" axis of the body. It is this composite invariant axis that becomes the base for the internal referential system that is then projected out into space.

Harmon felt that the work and illumination demands of our culture force us into persistent and prolonged postural skews which result in muscular tensions that eventually warp the invariant axis. This, in turn, results in spatial wraps and changes in actual spatial operation ability. In other words, to Harmon, the way we organize, interpret and act in space is derived from the way we ourselves are organized in terms of our internal, gravitationally based, coordinate systems.

Noting the effect that head and eye movements have on posture and, in turn, the effect that shifts in posture tend to have on head and eye position, Harmon concluded that vision and posture are highly interrelated. He felt, however, that because of the extensive postural demands of our culture, it is warped posture that triggers most of the visual problems that are encountered.

Harmon, however, was confronted with a number of enigmas. One was the fact that not everyone who demonstrated a persistent postural warp revealed a matching ocular effect. His first conclusion was that there is often a time lag involved during which period an organism acts "as if" a problem was present even though it has not yet affected structure. When asked to account for those who demonstrated decade(s)-long postural warps while still not manifesting concomitant visual changes; Harmon was compelled to conclude that, "If a postural warp causes a visual warp, then the two will be related. However, an ocular anomaly may have a different skew than the postural anomaly since the latter is not always responsible for the former...When the visual distortion is of long standing and has affected the postural position, the geometry of the postural skewing is not equal to the visual. However, when a body mechanic's mismatch has created a visual skewing, they will be similar geometrically."

A second, somewhat related, enigma that Harmon was confronted with had to do with refractive status. Harmon felt that the alignment of the vertical segments of the body related to refractive status while the positioning of the lateral segments of the body appeared to be related to phoria measurements. He specifically associated a persistent shifting of the center of gravity forward with myopia. A shift of the center of gravity forward also tends to cause the head to angle backwards (a chin up position) as part of the body's natural counterbalancing with gravity. Many individuals with a forward placed center of gravity, however, exhibit a chin down posture not only when they work but even when they are in an erect, posturally relaxed position. Harmon interprets this situation in an interesting way. He stated that "somebody acting like a myope will move his center of gravity towards the center of his near task, but if he is trying to preserve some hyperopic latitude, he will also alter the position of his head and shoulders. The top will look like he is pulling away and the bottom will look like he is moving in." In other words, Harmon acknowledged that it was possible for head posture to override trunk posture in determining refractive status. What he didn't pursue, however, were the elements involved in this override, the implication behind the phrase, "<u>trying</u> to preserve some hyperopic latitude."

Harmon also contributed the concept of orientation and localization.[5,6] Orientation, to Harmon, represented the establishment of a frame of reference so that an individual could know where he is in space in relation to the things in space. In other words, orientation, to Harmon, involved a relationship between an individual and his goal (a "me – it" type relationship). Localization, on the other hand, was viewed as involving locating the goal, determining what direction it was from the individual, and determining the relationship of one object in space with another (an "it – it" type relationship).

Harmon primarily conceived of orientation and localization as operational constructs. He felt that some individuals are better at and rely more upon one function than the other and that this preference, for example, would differentiate the myope from the hyperope. He only very generally discussed mechanisms for these functions. He considered orientation, for example, to be based on the interaction of the visual coordinate system with those body mechanisms related to coming to balance with gravity, predominantly the neural messages coming from the neck area (C2, C3, and C4). He considered that localization was related to "bilateral functioning...involving the two sides of the body...(which)...help determine our capacity to center and localize."[7]

Interestingly, Harmon's attributing the mechanism of orientation to proprioceptive information from the neck (C2, C3, and C4) is related directly to the work of Leonard Cohen.[8] Cohen did three experiments on monkeys. In one experiment, he surgically and/or chemically blocked the action of the extraocular muscles. In spite of this interpretation, the monkeys could still do tasks such as getting to and climbing a ladder to reach a trapeze. In a second experiment, he surgically and/or chemically blocked the inner ear mechanisms related to the labyrinths and accompanying ocular reflexes. In these instances, the monkeys could determine their relationship to the ladder when they stood still, but could not get to their destination once they started moving. They acted as if they knew where they were but could not locate their goal in space. In the third experiment, Cohen surgically and/or chemically blocked the proprioceptive fibers of the neck concerned with signals from the upper body. With this type of interference, the monkeys lost the ability to walk straight ahead. They could aim their eyes but acted as if they had no concept of the relationship to their goal. In other words, to Cohen, the monkeys lost their body orientation ability. It is for this reason that Harmon associated the term orientation with the upper cervical vertebrae.

It should be noted that the term orientation is used often with different connotations. Harmon, for example, used it at times as a noun to represent one's internal frame of reference and at other times as a verb to indicate how one operates in space. Cohen appeared to prefer the latter definition using terms like "body orientation" and "body spatial orientation" rather than the term "orientation" alone.

It is also possible to interpret the apparent aimless movement of the third group of monkeys in Cohen's experiment as being due to induced physiological mismatches among the mechanisms concerned with transport and manipulation rather than with that of orientation, per se. But, then, it all depends on how terms are defined.

A Psycho-Behavioral Approach
My own approach, a psycho-behavioral one, adds another dimension to the Harmon model. Where Harmon, for example, conceived of three organismic referential coordinate systems (the torso, head and visual system), my own philosophy considers that there is a fourth referential system, that one of individualized consciousness which establishes an internal mental map with the ego as its invariant canonical center.

Some of the components (or "coordinates") of this fourth "mental" referential system are spatial (parallel) processing, temporal (serial) processing, sensory imagery, language, primary experimental processing, symbolic processing, concrete processing, abstract processing, central processing, peripheral processing, logic, emotional feeling-tone, behavioral detachment and behavioral involvement mechanisms, etc., all operating around an ego which serves the purpose of stabilizing the mental field by acting as a mental "space center" or mental "spatial benchmark." The action of the ego, in turn, is organized around attitudes, beliefs, biases, and values through which the world is then interpreted.

The interaction of these four referential systems with consciousness that helps create an internal map that is projected out into space. With this map one develops the ability to judge one's self in space, relate to the things that are in space, relate things in space to each other, and to operate in space.

In addition, this internal map, biased by one's emotions, attitudes, values, beliefs, etc., also determines how one's physical mechanisms respond to situations including the flexibility or lack of it in returning to baseline normality either during or after an event.

Using the premise as a starting point, therefore, orientation and localization are viewed as mental constructs and not as mechanisms residing in any particular body part.

Orientation is seen as the attuning or aligning of consciousness towards or with a stimulus, object or event; as a directional mental movement towards what the organism wishes to attend. It is an act of basic conscious recognition (or interest) that something is out there.

Localization is seen as the process of establishing a relationship between one's self and what one wishes to attend, an act of mental triangulation between one's self as a bilateral organism and aspects of the environment. It entails a conscious "grasp" of what is recognized as being out there. In essence, therefore, both orientation and localization are seen as fundamental elements in the process of attention.

According to this view, orientation and localization are considered as being primarily mental constructs that are reflected in all aspects of behavior, visual as well as postural. In fact, it is how these constructs are organized around one's emotions and belief systems that influence who, for example, will act like a myope and become one and who will act like a myope and not become one. In addition, by placing the primary mechanisms for orientation and localization in the fourth consciousness-based coordinate referential system and not in any particular group of muscles, we can explain how an individual paralyzed from the neck down can still have adequate basic spatial orientation ability while exhibiting an inadequate or absent ability to move in space or manipulate objects.

This view also suggests that persistent refractive deviations, visuo-spatial warps as well as persistent rigid-type postural alternations are, more often than not, reflections of persistent attitudes, emotions, beliefs, biases, value judgments and self image.

This approach also leads to a slightly different interpretation of diagnostic information. Skeffington, for example, conceived of vision as being a spatial event and he viewed the analytical examination as probing how an individual structures his space world.[9] Harmon conceived of visual spatial action as being predominantly a reflection of how one's postural status and internal coordinate system relate to gravity and he, therefore, perceived the analytical examination as a means of probing the end results of one's postural status as it might be reflected in the visual system.

Those who hold a more physiologically oriented model of the visual process may accept the spatial and postural attributes of vision but feel more comfortable with the reflection of these actions in terms of accommodation and convergence mechanisms. For them, the analytical examination reveals what is happening within the accommodative-convergence systems as well as in the neural organization of these processes.

From the point of view that consciousness is the primary element in this interaction, the analytical examination is seen to reveal not only spatial, postural and accommodative-convergence elements but also the end result of one's biases, attitudes, self-image and basic belief systems through which one's space world and one's actions in space are structured.

This approach, therefore, envisions the psycho-spatial-visual-postural interaction as being multi-dimensional implying that persistent visual, perceptual, postural or psychological skews can affect each other. However, unlike Harmon who perceived that the major influence in the total organismic interaction is usually postural, this view stresses that, if priorities are to be assigned it is the psychological factor that appears to cast the major influence on all aspects of human function. In other words, this model considers the attributes of consciousness as being the organizing matrix for most of human and visual behavior.

It also suggests that a possible function of lenses and prisms may be to act as an indirect stimulus to change mental states through changes in internal computing which then secondarily result in an accompanying change in both ocular and postural states.

Harmon,[1] by the way, quoting Duke-Elder,[10] liked to stress the fact that 20% of the optic nerve fibers coming from the retina never get to the higher visual centers in the occipital lobe but go instead to the superior colliculus and then to the head and neck. Even though this was impressive to him, in terns of relating visual function to posture, what should be even more impressive is how little we know about the intricate interaction of the 80% of the optic nerve fibers that do go to the so called "higher centers" and how they, in turn are influenced by central control and "mental states."

The "mental states" factor has other interesting ramifications. It is a common observation, for example, that some individuals, regardless of age, demonstrate persistent residual visual and/or postural skews after completing a demanding near point visual task. Others, again, regardless of age, can work for hours in adverse visual and/or postural situations and be able to return to a fully relaxed and flexible visual and postural stance when the task is completed. The key element in what occurs appears to be due less to the potential "stressfulness" of the task than to the "rigidity" in one's approach to the task – one's psychological pre-set. The more rigid the approach the less the individual is able to maintain full and flexible operational degrees of freedom.

The rigidity of one's approach to a task, in turn, relates directly to one's "orientation" to that task. Orientation, as described earlier, refers to the "me-it" relationship. One aspect of this relationship is attitudinal in nature, mainly whether the "me-it" or "me versus it" ("me against it" or "it against me").

Therefore, the "containment" properties of a near visual task (as Skeffington saw it) or the postural skews induced by the physical surrounds such as improper seating and lighting (as Harmon saw it) may be stress-producing factors but the primary element in determining the degree of an individual's stress response and how he adapts, whether or not there is a loss of resiliency in function and whether or not there are permanent changes in structure, appears to be attitudinal. The effect, the primary element appears to be one's psychological "posture."

In other words, as one's attitudes and motives alter one's emotional "tonal" repertoire (his psycho-"logic"), an influence is then cast on both the individual's operational style (which includes his perceptual, cognitive, personality, and visual style) and also his bio-"logic" resulting in alterations in physiological function in both the autonomic (visceral) and somatic (skeletal) domains. It is this latter aspect which is then seen to affect such factors as accommodative-convergence relationships and postural status.

This view, therefore, comprises one element of my own personal "psycho-behavioral" approach to understanding visual function. I simply wished to share that with you here today.

References

1. Harmon DB. Notes on a Dynamic Theory of Vision, 3rd Rev. Austin, TX: Research Publications, 1958.
2. Grossfeld HD. Visual space and physical space. J Psychol 1951;32:25-33.
3. Harmon DB. Seminar Transcript, November, 1966.
4. Harmon DB. The rationale in development vision training. Seminar Transcript, March, 1966.
5. Harmon DB. Seminar Notes, May, 1969.
6. Harmon DB. Orientation and localization. Seminar Notes, September, 1969.
7. Harmon DB. Restrained performance as a contributing cause of visual problems. Optom Wkly 1966 Jul 7.
8. Cohen L. the role of eye and neck proprioceptive mechanisms in body orientation and motor coordination. J Neurophysiol 1961;24:1-11.
9. Skeffington, AM. Clinical applied optometry. Santa Ana, CA: Optometric Extension Program Postgraduate Papers, 1946-1973,
10. Duke-Elder W.S. Textbook of Ophthalmology, Vol. I., St. Louis:Mosby, 1946.

Zen and the Art of Vision Maintenance

Barry G. Millis, O.D.
Carlisle, PA

Maintaining one's vision is a revolutionary idea as described by the behavioral optometrist. First, we must expand the patient's knowledge of what vision is, and then hope he or she understands it well enough to follow through with the maintenance program of routine progress evaluations, control of environmental factors, and diligent use of plus lenses. The patient, in the office, listens attentively, responding enthusiastically to the behavioral mode and then goes home to family only to find that it is like trying to explain $E=Mc^2$. Actually, several years ago, I began occasionally saying to patients, "Behavioral optometry is like the shift from Newton's physics to Einstein's physics – there is a fundamental change in perspective."

I failed to recognize the full perspective myself until having read Fritjof Capra's, *The Turning Point*. Here is a physicist, the high priest of science, stating a powerful case for expanding scientific inquiry into areas long considered taboo such as the realm of subjective experience. Capra describes the development of the scientific method as used by Descartes and Newton. Their methods were derived from the concept that the universe is like a giant clockwork whose parts can be measured, analyzed, and categorized. This mechanistic viewpoint is today pervasive in all health sciences, biology, economics, and virtually anywhere you look. It is so much a part of the fabric of our lives that most of us do not realize that it is only one way of visualizing reality.

Additional perspective was found in Robert Pirsig's, *Zen and the Art of Motorcycle Maintenance*. He goes back further than Capra and shows how Descartes got turned on by the Greek trio of Socrates, Plato, and Aristotle. We are shown that this trio was in conflict with a school of thought that called for the integration of rational thinking with all other experience, but we know the outcome of that conflict.

Today we have a population that thinks of their bodies as an assemblage of parts that can go bad, at which time they go to a doctor to have the offending part repaired. The Cartesian model gives the physician rational support for treating disease as though it were independent of the patient and the patient was separate from the doctor.

Now the behavioral optometrist says to them, "You are a whole person and your eyes are but a small part of the process of vision." We say that, "Vision problems are caused by stress and the resultant eye defects are something you do to yourself." These words roll off our tongues, but do we realize the intellectual leap required to understand them. We are part of nothing less than a revolution in Western thought. The physicists have found that objective data is an illusion, that nothing exists independently of everything else, and that reality has a dynamic nature with no absolutes. As a behavioral optometrist, I readily understand these profound concepts that are unknown to most people. Actually, behavioral optometry has provided me with a means to share not only the leading edge of my profession, but to be at the vanguard of Western thought. The challenge is to be able to communicate these ideas to our patient, colleagues, and optometry students.

Behavioral optometry demands that we do nothing less than reorient our whole view of reality. Trying to understand the application of plus lenses, or the value of visual training within a Cartesian mentality is an effort doomed to result in frustration and denial. I have always found it impossible to write a report of a vision evaluation that even begins to encompass my experience of the interaction with the patient. When I write a report in the generally accepted manner it sounds far too analytical and logical. Most of our reports include phrases like "the child has an accommodative flexibility problem" or "the patient has a binocularity problem" as though these phrases describe cause-effect relationships. While it is true that we see these areas of difficulty, I believe it does our profession a disservice to couch our observations in Cartesian terminology that only reduces our beautifully dynamic, holistic concepts to artificial categories.

A good example of the intellectual conflict that exists even with behavioral optometry is the reaction to a statement that Robert A. Kraskin made, "We train people not findings." A practitioner with Cartesian ears gets uncomfortable with decisions not based on numbers, in spite of the fact that the numbers are not relevant. I doubt most ODs would consider a refractive status of -3.50 D a successful myopia control case when the patient started wearing plus as an emmetrope. Yet if one is concerned with the whole person and recognizes that in the primary myope unstable visual space is primarily a reflection of an insecure ego, then the control of the ocular manifestation will take time. We are not talking about controlling eyeballs, but rather changing a person's self-image. To base success strictly on numbers is restrictive and unrealistic. If our goal is only the narrow one of a distance subjective (#7) in plus, then the more general goal of dynamic balance between positive and self-defeating behavior remains untouched. With ongoing therapy in the form of bifocals and periods of visual training, eventually the apparently uncontrolled myope returns to the office reporting that his or her lenses are too strong while the parents report substantial positive changes in attitude. All that guidance and talk of effortless processing has finally been assimilated.

If we consider myopia to be the end result of an adaptive process in response to various stresses focused at nearpoint, does the time spent in transition from emmetropia to myopia represent a restriction of function with associated restrictions in thinking? Does myopia control have value primarily because of the maintenance of flexible function rather than simply preventing the loss of distance acuity? We can say that wearing lenses to compensate for myopia is not so terrible and that myopia control is not all that important, but that the restriction of function during the adaptive process is the main problem. The visual behavior that is repeated and reinforced to the level of habit has lasting impact on the function of a myopic person long after the visual pattern has stabilized and organized. The inability of many myopes to be aware of the intensity of their effort has ramifications in everything they do. One may say that myopia allows an individual to deal more easily with near-centered tasks, but I think that position ignores the process of myopia and only considers the refractive end-point.

Over the last few years I have grown increasingly uncomfortable with the way we differentiate between functional and pathological disorders. We believe that functional ocular defects like myopia, astigmatism, and adverse hyperopia are manifestations of underlying stress. In Capra's *The Turning Point*, he writes that, "Excessive stress is believed to contribute significantly to the origin and development of most diseases, manifesting itself in the organism's initial imbalance and, subsequently, being channeled through a particular personality configuration to give rise to specific disorders." Lewis Thomas in *The Lives of a Cell* writes, "Inflammation is caused by the body's overreaction to an invading organism." Is not myopia the body's overreaction to invading culture?

There is a difference between illness and disease that corresponds to our differentiation between visual stress syndrome and the end-point ocular defect. If one views all illness as part of the same process, what are the implications for visual training?

In Eastern traditions, health is considered part of the dynamic ebb and flow of life, with no expectation of perpetual freedom from illness. Indeed, illness can serve the useful purpose of guiding us to use our finite energy wisely. The goal in Cartesian thinking is to eliminate disease by chemically destroying those pesky invaders that are part of nature's war against us. The Eastern philosophies consider disease to be the end result of disharmony in one's life or overall life style. This concept extends to diseases of the whole society as well. We are not at war with nature unless we make the declaration. In visual training could we not aid an individual to be more aware and sensitive to his own dynamic flow? We happen to see people whose personality configuration and environmental interaction has produced visual illness, but by being more peripheral could we not teach then to generalize the process learned in VT to illness of all kinds? The boundaries of optometry are infinite. Therapeutic drugs are child's play.

What excited me about Capra's book is the breadth and depth of the revolution of which we are a part. It is apparent that in all fields of economic, social, health, and hard sciences we must utilize holistic, dynamic models for greater understanding. Capra, the physicist tells us that a science does not need to have quantifiable, so-called objective data. Indeed, meaning is lost by attempting to squeeze all of reality into statistical cubbyholes. Visual training is the obvious example. The often heard criticism that we do not have "hard data" to support our work begins to lose relevance. Much of what occurs in visual training is subjective, and instead of wavering, we must be willing to include subjective experience as a legitimate part of reality. This is not a condemnation of logical analysis, but rather a request for balance. Actually, the dynamic nature of things assures that the holistic frame of mind will ascend to command our attention.

Then eventually as exceptions and questions impossible to ignore overload the system, there will be a shift back to the rational side. Continual ebb and flow, left brain-right brain, Yin and Yang, and with each oscillation both sides are enhanced as the textures become more varied and complex. Subjective experience means something very different to us than to medieval men and women. We are, after all, children of a time when rational analysis flexed its muscles and set a torrid pace. We openly accept the gifts of rational accomplishment but urge the reasoning mind to shed its amblyopia toward those things beyond logic. I urge you all to consider the Art of Vision Maintenance for its esthetic value – the view is sublime this time of year.

Bibliography
Capra F. The Turning Point: Science, Society, and the Rising Culture. New York:Bantam Doubleday Dell, 1988. ISBN: 0553345729
Thomas L. The Lives of a Cell.
Pirsig R. Zen and the Art of Motorcycle Maintenance. Bantam Books, 1982. ISBN: 0553207083

Involuntary Focus and Convergence at the Resting State of the Human Eye

Ronald Shane, O.D.
Sunbury, PA

Visual perception involves the recognition and localization of objects in space. The human visual system does not always accomplish these tasks efficiently. It appears that the ability to identify objects as well as accurately locate them depends heavily on both the conditions of observation as well as individual visual traits. Why is it that some people see better than others under adverse conditions when both are fully corrected or need no refractive correction as measured by conventional standards? This challenging statement may soon be answered with the help of vision scientists like Dr. Fred Owen and Dr. Hershel Leibowitz, who have advanced the field of knowledge on the resting state of the human eye.

Present clinical refractive techniques reveal visual abnormalities as measured under the conditions of testing or normal conditions. We rarely test patients under adverse or stressful conditions to obtain a distance correction. Realistically, all practicing optometrists have had many patients who acted adversely to the given spectacle prescription when attempting to utilize them in the real world. Further attempts to resolve their problem led to greater frustration for both the doctor and patient. The patient may try several eye doctors without finding a satisfactory pair of glasses, or might get lucky and receive a prescription that suits their needs better. When examining that 'best pair of glasses I ever had' we find the RX to be incompatible with our findings, and it either overcorrected or undercorrected, but the patient loves them.

The answers to some of these puzzling cases probably involve many factors, such as the patient's sensitivity to spatial contrast, previous experience, ability to concentrate on a given task, and tolerance of physiological and psychological stress, along with other unknown factors. These many factors may interact in ways that defy prediction. Recent research does indicate that visual perception under adverse conditions can be seriously limited by both the accommodative and ocular-motor systems. These limitations can be predicted by simple tests and compensation can be made with lenses.

Visual scientists began serious studies on the resting state of the human eye about 12 years ago. Those studies revealed systematic biases that come into play under adverse conditions. Further research revealed a variety of perceptual problems that are explainable and even negated by corrective lenses. Drs. Owens and Leibowitz soon realized the implications of their research toward solving problems encountered in the real world. The major insight from this research revolves around the phenomenon that occurs whenever visual conditions are degraded. The eyes tend to shift involuntarily to the subject's resting distance, which varies widely on an individual basis and frequently is not appropriate for viewing object distance. Under these circumstances, the resting state can hinder both the object recognition and the accuracy of spatial perception.

Adler states myopes with high refractive errors complain of night blindness and show raised thresholds of dark adaptation. He states this is more prevalent in myopes above 5 diopters. He further states that no good explanation for this association has yet been given.
Borish states Lord Ragleigh is generally credited with noting this existence of night blindness, but the actual first mention of this anomalous myopia dates back to Nevil Maskelyne, who stated his celestial observations were clearer when viewing through concave lenses. He noted that those same lenses offered no help in bright illumination. He also established the existence of the chromatic aberration in the eye which he measured at 0.535 mm.

The next author of this anomaly, William Kitchiner, estimated his night myopia at 0.31 Diopter. Luckiesh, Moss and Reese, whose studies in 1937 and 1939 respectively, found -0.75 D change to be the most frequent, followed by -0.50 D, with only 12.4% of the subjects exhibiting night myopia.

Knoll, in 1952, attributed night myopia to the following:
    Spherical aberrations.
    Obliquity.
    Chromatic aberration.
    Accommodation.
    Adaptation and retinal luminance distribution

He sums up with the following causes:
Spherical alleviation, which increases as the pupil dilates.
Chromatic aberration and the Purkinje shift.
A true far point, far resting accommodation, within infinity, allied to the accommodative status of empty space.

Richards, in 1967, offers the following advice. Vision is usually at the mesopic, not scotopic, levels, down to 0.0003 f.1.[1] during night driving. At this range, the Purkinje shift may create 0.10 D myopia. When the pupil dilated from 4 to 7.5 mm this shift may increase from 0.20 D to as much as 1.00 D of myopia. He found only 20% of his subjects gained increased acuity with added minus. Most were emmetropic.

Borish further states that if no stimulus is presented to the eye as in the absence of light or in low illumination, accommodation does not reach a point of "neutrality." The eye becomes more myopic as luminance is reduced and at very low levels, becomes about 2.00 D more myopic (Alpern and David 1958). Young adults were found not to relax accommodation beyond 2 m and to lag in the amount of accommodation up to 1 m (Graft 1953). Alpern and Larson noted the recession of the near point and that the far point moved closer. The ACA ratio remained constant but with a reduced amplitude. Heath (1956) stated nocturnal myopia to be from 1.50 D to 1.75 D. He stated tonus, convergence, nearness and blurredness are all contributing factors.

Morgan (1967) states accommodation may be in a resting state when night myopia is exhibited, the same being true for empty field myopia. He postulated that if no blur stimulus was present, chromic accommodation was active.

Borish again states that during scotopic vision there is a shift towards myopia, known as night myopia. With luminance below 1 flux, the maximum sensitivity of the eye shifts from 550 to 510 millimicrons.
Research during World War II seems to indicate that the above explanations fail to explain why some subject's show as much as 4.00 D of night myopia, while others under the exact same conditions exhibited none at all. With the range of pupil size not exceeding 5 mm,

---

[1] *f.1. refers here to the f-stop equivalent as used to classify the light transmissibility of camera lenses or optical system. For reference purposes this unit is approximately 16 times more light-sensitive than an f2.8 lens, which is standard on most single lens reflexes.*

the changes in optical aberrations and spectral sensitivity should not be so great among individuals. Certainly the pupil size fails to become a factor in space myopia when viewing a bright empty field, or when using optical instruments in instrument myopia.

In the early 1970s, the laser optometer provided a new tool for studying accommodation. The unique characteristic of the laser's interference is that is allows precise measurements of the eye's focus without stimulating changes in accommodation. A new era of research was initiated.

The laser optometer offered the first convenient, as well as accurate, technique for measuring the resting focus of the eyes. The use of this instrument gave proof to the abandoned theory of the eyes focusing at an intermediate distance in darkness. On a small project involving 220 college students, Owens and Leibowitz showed the mean dark focus value was about 1.50 D (67 cm). All the subjects were fully corrected and wore their glasses during testing or were emmetropes. The data obtained indicated that the subjects varied widely in the value of their dark focus. The range of dark focus varied 4.00 D to Plano. Only 1% of the subjects focused at optical infinity. There was no apparent relationship between the refractive error and the resultant dark focus. The authors then speculated that perhaps all anomalous "myopias" were due to a passive shift of accommodation toward its resting state, therefore, indicating that different persons are likely to exhibit different levels of anomalous myopia, depending on their idiosyncratic dark-focus values.

Leibowitz and Owens, in 1975, ran a series of studies, testing whether the dark-focus could be used to predict the severity of anomalous myopias. In a very small study the dark-focus was compared with the focus when viewing a distant residential scene at different levels of illumination. As the luminescence was varied from full daylight to values similar to a moonlit night, the accuracy of the accommodative system deteriorated. Most subjects became increasingly myopic with reduced luminance. The night myopia ranged from 0.5 D to 2.5 D. The results were carefully matched with the subject's dark focus and the results clearly showed that the subjects who had a near dark-focus had proportionally greater night myopia that those with a far dark-focus.

The above findings tend to indicate that anomalous myopias are not refractive errors in the clinical sense, since they really are not the results of anatomical defects intrinsic to the eye. They are focusing errors that result from normal variations in the behavior of accommodation. Under stressful or degraded conditions the eyes can no longer change focus efficiently while the individual's resting focus is not ideally suited for visual tasks.

The question of what, exactly, is being degraded under deteriorating conditions has not been determined by researchers in this field. Certainly the loss of luminance is itself not the singular answer since similar myopic responses occur in bright illumination. Owens hypothesized that to control the eye's focus, the brain required data on the contrast of the retinal image. When this data is insufficient, the accommodation tends to remain near the individual's dark-focus. As the stimulus is degraded, the accommodative attempt to focus the image has progressively less effect on its retinal contrast so that the range of distance over which accommodation operates progressively diminishes. Most subjects showed a bias toward an intermediate focal distance, resulting in myopia at far while increasing hyperopia for near objects.

The following charts by Owens illustrate:

Near Dark Focus (3.5D)

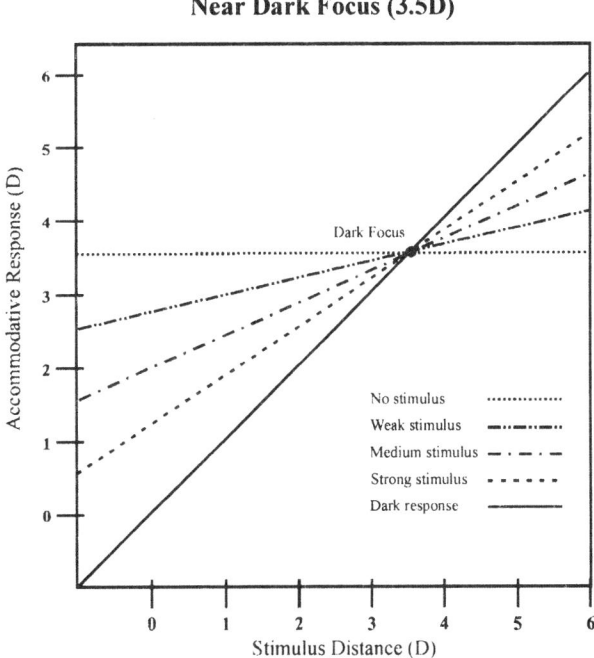

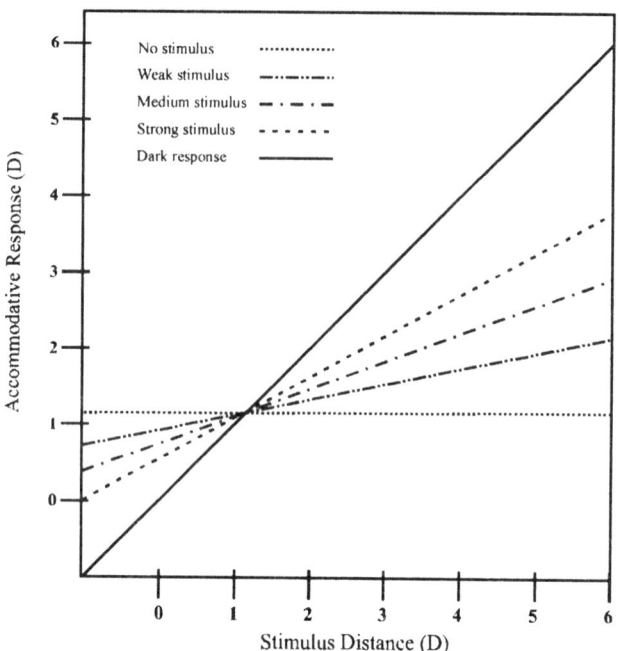

Far Dark Focus (1.0D)

The charts show that when visual conditions deteriorate, the individual with an intermediate resting focus tends to become myopic for distant objects and hyperopic for close objects. The graph on the left shows the response of a subject with a near dark-focus; on the right, a subject with a far dark-focus. In both cases, accurate accommodation would produce a line with unit slope, since the focal distance would match the target distance in every instance. As conditions deteriorate, responses move toward a line with a slope of zero. The eyes tend more and more to remain at their resting focus, regardless of the distance to the target. Note that the eye always accommodates accurately for the objects at the individual's idiosyncratic dark-focus distance. The accommodation is always accurate, regardless of stimulus quality for targets position at the distance of the observer's focus (Johnson 1976). Therefore, the accuracy of accommodation, which determines the clarity of the retinal image, depends on two general factors; the quality of the visual stimuli; and the distance of the stimulus to the observer's dark-focus.

Leibowitz and Owens are of the opinion that all anomalous myopias result from a loss of sensory feedback about the effect of accommodation on the retinal image. If this interpretation is correct, it should be possible to predict and correct anomalous myopias on the basis of the dark-focus. Leibowitz and Owens (1976) performed two studies to prove their hypothesis. The first involved both lab and field-testing of refractive correction for night driving. The preliminary experiment involved measured accommodation for a simulated road sign presented at varying luminance and contrast levels typical of those encountered on the highway at night. The results showed most subjects focused approximately halfway between the distant sign and their individual dark-focus, suggesting that a myopic correction of one-half the dark focus power would improve visibility during night driving. This finding was confirmed subjectively in field tests in which the subjects were given three sets of unlabeled spectacles to compare under night driving conditions. All the subjects preferred the half dark-focus correction to their normal daytime and full dark-focus corrections. In addition, some subjects stated this half dark-focus correction reduced the eye-strain and general fatigue associated with night driving. My own findings under office testing, utilizing test letters at 20 ft. and varying lighting conditions indicated optimum minus was closer to -0.37 D. I could not lower the illumination in the room to simulate the most severe conditions found in the real environment. After three minutes with the darkest illumination I could establish, both shape and edge detecting became apparent, which some patients did utilize as visual clues.

Owens states it is important to remember that although he found that subjects preferred the half the dark-focus lenses to general night driving, these lenses may not be optimal for all low-visibility conditions. Signs, traffic and road markings within the headlights' illumination provided some spatial contrast to guide accommodation, resulting in focusing responses that fall between the ideal adjustment and the individual's dark-focus. In these situations greater minus would be optimal.

Owens tested the above theory for empty-field myopia by measuring detection thresholds for a tiny (1.0 mm) bright point of light superimposed on a uniform background showed the greatest sensitivity when using the full dark-focus correction; and the degree that his correction enhanced their performance depended on each subject's dark-focus. When the threshold of visibility was related to monograms that predict aircraft sighting ranges, increases in sighting range varied from 26% for a subject with a relatively distant dark-focus (0.1 D) to 316% for one with a relatively near dark-focus (2.0 D). Luria, in 1980, duplicated these findings, suggesting that the ability of some pilots to detect aircraft and other small stimuli could be improved by a spectacle correction that cannot be obtained by standard refractive techniques.

The "Mandelbaum effect" seems to relate to the dark-focus phenomenon. Studies show that the distance of maximum interference corresponds to the observer's dark focus. The relationship of the windshield distance from the driver or pilot and their dark-focus could produce serious visual impairment due to myopic accommodation for rain, dirt, scratches, reflected headlights and other image formations on the windshield.

There is evidence to substantiate the belief that visual performance on near tasks depends on the individual's dark focus. Can we then utilize the dark focus in prescribing the near Rx or add? It has been shown that video display users who have a near dark-focus usually can focus more accurately and suffer less fatigue than those with a far dark-focus (both being fully corrected for their distant refractive error). Some research has indicated that acuity is optimal at the observer's dark-focus for people who initially have a far resting position. Further research is necessary to correlate progressive myopia with the inward shift of the dark-focus.

The Mandelbaum effect can be utilized to estimate the dark-focus in your office with very little expense. I use a mesh window screen and raise the level of the exam chair so that the patients' eye level is equal to the acuity chart. I utilize the 20/20 and 20/25 line with the patient's habitual glasses on. While the patient is fixating the line, I place the screen in the line of sight near the chart. I then move toward the observer slowly constantly asking if the letters are readable. When the patient states he cannot distinguish the letters, I stop, remove the screen for comparison, and then re-introduce the screen. If the patient still cannot read the letters when the screen is reintroduced, then I measure that distance in meters from the patient. I redo the test, starting from the patient, and moving backward toward the acuity chart. Again, confirm the blur by comparing with the screen removed. This should closely match the distance of the previously obtained reading. I take readings in full illumination and in the darkened room. The reciprocal of the distance in meters will approximate the dark-focus calculation.
While I am holding the screen at the dark-focus distance, I ask the patient to place minus lenses before both eyes and tell me when the letters are restored to sharpness. When this is done under reduced

illumination, you now have the approximate correction for use at night or in equally reduced illumination. The amount of minus will change as the edge clues and forms clues are eliminated.

The second aspect of importance in dealing with vision under reduced illumination is space perception. Early on, Descartes proposed that accommodation and vergence could be used to determine the distance of fixated objects. Philosophers like George Blakely, speculated that distance perception is learned through the association of sensory experience and binocular vergence. Much research over the past 30 years confirms that both accommodation and vergence affect space perception, more so at near. Recent research indicates the accuracy of distance perception is variable and degenerates rapidly when visual clues are removed from the visual field. It seems that localization errors reflect a bias toward an intermediate distance. This would explain why most people underestimate the distance of objects at far, while overestimating near objects under visual stressful conditions.

Gogel and colleagues extensively studied this specific distance tendency. He demonstrated that objects are consistently localized at an intermediate distance whenever extrinsic distance information is eliminated. He found a wide variation in specific distance tendency, ranging between 30cm, to over 8m, with the average approximately 2m. This perceived error is true of object size, motion, and distance. Gogel's explanation suggests an individual's specific distance represents a fundamental metric of perceived space and therefore, influences perception under a wide range of conditions. This would mean that the specific distance tendency might prove to be a key variable for predicting a person's ability to localize objects in space.

The classic example of specific distance tendency is the illusion of the moon's variable size. When near the horizon, the moon appears larger than when seen at its zenith. The moon at its zenith is unconsciously perceived to be nearer than when close to the horizon. The apparently nearer zenith moon seems smaller than the apparently farther horizon moon.

When extrinsic information is reduced, the phenomenon of systematic distortion of perceived space occurs. New evidence indicates accommodation is biased toward an intermediate distance when under reduced illumination can be related with specific distance tendency. If the visual involvement is reduced in clues so that extrinsic distance information is eliminated, then we can assume that intrinsic factors such as oculomotor adjustments will be used to determine the perceived distance. If those oculomotor adjustments are biased toward their intermediate resting state, as shown by Leibowitz, then the perceived distance should show a correlated bias toward the same intermediate distance.

Owens and Leibowitz showed that both the apparent distance and accommodation were biased toward an intermediate distance, with mean values of 145cm for the specific distance tendency and 51cm for the dark-focus. No significant correlation was established between the specific distance tendency and the dark-focus. Fincham had reported that accommodation and vergence disassociated in darkness. He found in the absence of retinal images both responses tended to shift toward different resting positions. Owens and Leibowitz compared binocular vergence and distance perception under low illumination. The phoria was measured in darkness to obtain the resting position of vergence. The measure was referred to as the 'dark vergence' and indicated the distance for which the eyes fixated when there are no visible stimuli. This value was compared with the perceived distance of a single point of light viewed under the same dark conditions. They found a systematic relationship. The apparent distance of the point of light was highly correlated with the subject's dark vergence. Those people with a near dark vergence underestimated the distance more than those with a far dark vergence position. This would indicate that the specific distance tendency is related to the resting state of binocular vergence. If this is true, then perhaps other illusions of spatial perception may be predictable on the basis of each individual's dark vergence position.

Leibowitz and Owens feel that vergence and accommodation lose their well-known synergy and return to relatively independent resting positions under reduced stimulation. A second study by Leibowitz shows the average dark vergence and dark-focus values to be significantly different, with the mean dark vergence corresponding to 116cm. and the mean dark-focus at 76cm. He theorizes that both the dark-focus and the dark vergence appear to represent fundamental, yet different, characteristics of the oculomotor system's ability to deal with the third dimension.

Post and Leibowitz have also shown that compensatory eye movements, which normally stabilize a retinal image during head movements, tend to induce a 'slippage' of fixation for objects viewed in darkness at distances nearer or farther than the dark vergence distance. This tendency to lose fixation during head movements is counteracted by persistent movements of the eyes that eliminate retinal slip, but such pursuit causes the stationary object to appear to be moving. For objects beyond the dark vergence distance, the eyes must pursue in the same direction as the head movement to maintain fixation. For objects nearer than the dark vergence distance, the eyes must pursue in the direction opposite the head movement. In both cases the fixated object appears to move in the same direction as the pursuit effort required to eliminate the retinal slip. When the stimulus lies at the same distance as the dark vergence, no illusory motion is perceived.

What is of importance to the optometrist is the concept of loss of binocular fusion being the earliest and most devastating effect of psychological stress on visual performance. It has already been shown that hypoxia produces increased vergence errors and diplopia in pilots at altitudes. Stress producers such as hypoxia, alcohol, barbiturates, and other drugs initiate a progressive decrease in the operating range of binocular vergence. Initially, these people under the above stress seem to exhibit an over-convergence for distant stimuli and under-convergence for near stimuli. Greater stress produces greater fixation disparities at both far and near, leaving binocular fusion possible only for objects at some intermediate distance. We can then state that stress has the same effect on binocular vergence as reduced stimuli. Both conditions reduce the efficiency of those mechanics that control vergence with the response being biased toward the intermediate posture as shown by Owens and Leibowitz in 1983. The dark vergence position has not been experimentally compared to the vergence figures obtained with hypoxia and alcoholic intoxication. If some correlation exists then it will be possible to predict the effects of visual stress on an individual basis.

With the research showing that many forms of stress have direct bearing on both the accommodative and vergence system, the optometrist who encounters problem patients can now deal with this common problem in a more rational way. It would be most prudent for the optometrist who has a patient under great emotional stress to either postpone giving the Rx obtained under those conditions, or to re-schedule the patient for a second exam when they are under better control, since focusing behavior may depend on emotional arousal and personality as well as the quality of the stimulus.

Summary

The purpose of this paper is to make optometrists aware that research on the resting state of the eyes has provided surprising and useful insights into normal variations of visual performance. When visual conditions are degraded, the accommodation and binocular vergence become progressively biased toward an intermediate adjustment, regardless of the patient's refractive error. The "resting status" of accommodation and vergence are quantitatively different and vary widely on an individual basis.

Perceptual abilities are directly affected by the associated distortions. The dark focus of accommodation produces anomalous refractive errors such as night myopia, space myopia, and instrument myopia, as well as creating the Mandelbaum effect.

Most important to clinicians is the ability to nullify the problems created by dark-focus with appropriate lens changes.
Bias toward the dark vergence position gives rise to error of distance perception and may be responsible for those illusions involving size, motion, and localization.

Further research is needed to clarify the many problems and questions involving the above phenomenon and how they relate to physiological stress, age, and psychological stress.

By utilizing new techniques such as computer-assessed photo-refraction, infrared eye tracking, and other space-age instruments, new investigative data can be obtained with the absence of restraints of position and environment. This data may very well change the present concepts of how to correct for refractive errors and reinforce the concept of no "one prescription prescribing" to satisfy the needs of most people.

Bibliography
Adler, FH. Physiology of the Eye. St. Louis:C.V.Mosby, 1950.
Borish IM. Clinical Refraction 3rd ed. Chicago:The Professional Press, 1975:

Visual Imagery and the Plateau Spiral in Myopia Control

Elliott B. Forrest O.D., FAAO, FCOVD
New York, NY

As far back as the 1940s, a number of key vision training procedures were popular for myopia control. Outside of the Skeffington approach to lens application and the use of prism as recommended by Ray Morse-Peckham, the major therapeutic approaches for myopia control aimed at improving ocular motility skills, fusion ranges, accommodative flexibility, plus acceptance and tachistoscopic blur interpretation. An interesting adjunct technique that was also in vogue in the 1940s involved the use of the Plateau Spiral.

The Plateau Spiral received its name because of the initial work of Joseph Plateau, a Belgian psychophysicist who described in 1850 how observing a rotating arithmetic (Archimedes) spiral would result in the perception of a reversed aftereffect. If the spiral was viewed as rotating inwards toward its center, the perceived-after-effect when one's gaze was redirected elsewhere (toward objects or letters in space) would be an expansion or enlargement of what was being viewed, making smaller details more discernible. The opposite perceived after-effect would occur if the spiral was viewed as expanding outwards from its center. Some visual scientists considered that this effect was due to eye movements as the track of the spiral was followed. Others considered that it was due to retinal adaptation since the effect also seemed to be achieved when fixation was kept on only one localized area of the moving spiral. Still others, noting that the effect could be transferred to a previously occluded eye, felt that higher cortical processes were also involved.

Optometrists who used this technique found that it was quite dramatic from the patient's point of view; enabling letters to be read that were unreadable only moments before. It was assumed by many that using this procedure might ultimately lead to improved blur recognition, relaxed accommodation and reduced myopia. Practically however, the aftereffect was usually of short duration and did not appear to either increase overall blur interpretation or reduce myopia. It stimulated and motivated the patient but other procedures such as accommodative rock and plus acceptance seemed to be more directly related to either increased visual acuity or to actual refractive change. In 1967, T.W. White attempted to probe the possible relaxing effect of the rotating Plateau Spiral on accommodation and found no "appreciable alteration in accommodative responses." Unfortunately, White only utilized two subjects, both hyperopic rather than myopic, and investigated accommodative status using a retinoscope and haploscope while the subjects viewed the rotating spiral and not when they were experiencing the aftereffect.

A personal approach

Based on clinical experience, my early enthusiasm for the Plateau Spiral as a possible effective technique in myopia control waned over the years. I began to use it sparingly and mainly as a dramatic interlude for the patient rather than with the expectation that it would actually reverse myopia. My interest, however, was renewed about eight or nine years ago as I became involved with the subject of visual imagery and saw a way to use imagery to develop a novel and more fruitful method of applying the Plateau Spiral principle. The following is a summary of the key steps involved in this imagery approach:

1. The basic procedure starts in a traditional manner. The myopic patient is asked to observe a near or far Snellen chart to determine the lowest line that can be read comfortably. This is done without correction. The patient is then instructed to view a Plateau Spiral at a distance of between 16 to 30 inches, depending on the size of the spiral used. The spiral is slowly rotated so that it spins inwards toward its center with the patient being asked to experience the spiral as not only contracting inwards but to sense it going backwards in space as if it were a "time tunnel." This is done for approximately 60 to 90 seconds, after which the instruction is given to look back quickly at the near or far target and note if smaller letters can now be read. With repetition, the patient is encouraged to try to consciously maintain the after-effect for longer periods of time.

2. The second stage of this procedure is to have the patient view a stationary, non-rotating spiral and mentally follow the line of the spiral inward while imagining that it is both rotating toward its center and also floating outwards in space. As the after-effect is achieved with the stationary spiral, the patient is again encouraged to try to maintain the effect for as long as possible.

3. The third and most important step involves the active use of visual imagery in the absence of an actual stimulus. At this stage, it is

important to determine if reasonable basic visual imagery ability exists and whether it can be controlled. This is done by asking the patient to sit with eyes closed and picture an airplane, first seeing it flying forwards and then backwards; seeing a chair, a cat next to it and then seeing the cat jumping onto the chair; seeing an apple being bitten into and then seeing a worm (or half a worm) crawling out of the bitten part. Doing this reveals whether the patient has the ability to conjure up static visual images and whether image action can also be selfgenerated. This ability is an essential prerequisite for this stage which requires the patient to sit before the near or far letter chart with eyes closed and simply visualize a rotating spiral that occupies the full field of vision and to image it vividly contracting inwardly and moving outwardly like a "time tunnel." After maintaining this vivid visual image for at least 60 to 90 seconds, the eyes are opened and the extent and duration of the succeeding after-effect is noted as well as the patient's ability to read smaller letters. This step is then practiced until the achieved after-effect can be increased in magnitude and can occur more easily and effortlessly.

4. The last stage of this procedure involves practicing visualizing a rotating spiral with eyes open while the gaze is simultaneously directed at the near or far target. As this can be achieved, instructions are given to decrease the time the spiral is imaged as rotating while trying to hold onto the perceived after-effect. Finally, as efficiency is developed, the patient is encouraged to practice this open-eye imagery technique anytime, anywhere and anyplace better vision is needed. It could be while watching television, when observing a scoreboard at a ball game, while trying to read license plates or street signs when driving, while attempting to read the time on a clock across the room or when trying to copy from the blackboard in class. Some even reach the point of being able to self-generate the enlargement after-effect while bypassing the need to first image the inwardly contracting spiral.

The value of this technique is that it provides the myopic individual with a tool to voluntarily increase distance discrimination ability whenever it is needed. With practice, it tends to become more spontaneous, automatic and rapid. There have also been indications that this procedure alone may have a positive effect on refractive status. Although this aspect interests the optometrist, for the patient the ability to discriminate and identify more easily at will, has a tremendous practical value in and of itself.

The enigma of the circular disc
The following anecdote is only indirectly related to using the imaged Plateau Spiral procedure, yet it adds an interesting dimension to both the technique and the subject of myopia.

In the past decade I have been a proponent of what I have come to call a psycho-behavioral approach to visual function. One tenet of this philosophy favors the view that, for the most part, we are active participants in the selective adaptive outcomes (such as myopia) that so many of us end up with. In other words, this outlook suggests that we are highly involved in creating what we are and what we become, visually or otherwise. Based on this approach, one major direction in therapy is to attempt to set the stage for patients to begin to experience, whenever possible, that they have somehow, in some way and to some degree participated in the origin of their motility, binocular, accommodative or refractive difficulties and then to begin to experience that the ability to change and improve their status also rests with themselves: that they are in charge of both their vision and their lives. With this in mind, the following story becomes more powerful in its implications.

I was engaged in conversation with a young man in a non-optometric situation. In the course of our discussion, he mentioned that he was myopic and did not like it. I suggested that, if he were interested and wanted to try an "experiment," I would show him a technique that, if it worked, might control his vision and let him see better, at least on a temporary basis. He was enthusiastic about trying. Since he turned out to be a good imager, I went directly to the third stage of this procedure. He first looked across the room to determine what detail he could and could not see clearly. Then, sitting in a relaxed position he was instructed to "let go," close his eyes and picture a giant spiral "time tunnel" rotating slowly in toward its center while receding as if it were a giant cylinder going further and further into the distance. He was told to try to see this moving three-dimensional image so clearly and realistically that he would feel it was possible to physically go into it. He was also instructed to maintain this dynamic image until I told him to open his eyes at which time he was to look across the room and note if doing the procedure helped him see any better.

He closed his eyes and started to image the spiral. After about two minutes I asked him how he was doing. He replied that he was experiencing a somewhat disturbing phenomenon and wanted to stay with it a little longer. After approximately four or five minutes, with a look of relief and excitement on his face, he opened his eyes. I will try to reconstruct what he said to me as accurately as I can.

"I must tell you what happened," he said. "I was vividly imagining a giant slowly rotating 'time tunnel' as you told me to do and seeing it recede off into the distance. For some reason however, I just could not get to see the farthest end of the spiral. About three quarters of the way into the 'time tunnel' there appeared to be a circular gray disc that blocked my view and no matter how I tried or how long I worked at it I just could not get it to disappear. At first it was upsetting. Then as I thought about it, I began to recognize that since I was the one who was visualizing and creating the spiral in my mind, I must also be the one creating the gray disc that was blocking my vision. I was perplexed by this, when suddenly I realized that the persistent presence of that circular obstruction must represent my not actually wanting to see far away. It seems that although I vehemently dislike being nearsighted, at some deeper level I must want to be nearsighted otherwise I would not be setting up any blocks. Some part of me obviously does not want to deal with things off in the distance."

To alleviate this sense of frustration in not getting past his circular disc, I suggested a few possible ways the problem might be solved. However, the essence of our discussion developed into how one, in general, could get around or through all sorts of impasses, whether they occur in one's thoughts, one's visualizations or in one's everyday sensory-motor experiences. I also told him that he had undergone a very profound insight and that, in my opinion, this insight was one of the truly important steps in getting to the root of what functional myopia was all about.

I cannot guarantee that this type of spontaneous recognition will ever happen to anyone imaging a Plateau Spiral again but it was an exciting extension of using the imaging procedure. At the least, it resulted in my learning to ask other questions to those using the imaged spiral technique such as whether they can see the entire spiral, whether any part disappears or seems to be blocked, or whether anything appears to be unusual in any way. It is only as more appropriate questions begin to be asked that more revealing responses surface and often it only takes one insightful patient or one insightful interaction to open the door to new perspectives.

The Use of Base-Down Prism in the Treatment of the Cerebral Palsied Patient

Wendy C. Garson, O.D.
McLean, VA

For many years optometrists have been asked why certain procedures work, or why does a particular lens produce given results. Oftentimes, the response is that, "Whatever it is, it works, therefore don't question why." For some of us the reply was, "Physicians don't know how aspirin works and they keep prescribing it." Well, for a few years now some of the mode of action of aspirin has been known. The fact that aspirin's mode of action was unknown up until recently did not stop its use – but it also isn't stopping the search for a more complete answer. Behavioral optometry should take note of this in talking to other functionally oriented professionals such as physical and occupational therapists. We should not talk only of the art of optometry but also be able to make hypotheses based on a sound knowledge of science and physiology.

This paper is one such attempt to address a question that has bothered me for several years. The question is, why does a base-down prism improve trunk and head/neck control in a patient with cerebral palsy (CP)? On first looking at the picture, on would think that base-down prism would hinder instead of help the development of movement abilities. Unlike the hyperope, the center of gravity is often in front of the patient who has CP. Typically, the head posture of the hyperope is with the chin tucked, a flattened neck curve, hypotonicity in the neck and lower back, and possibly a posterior pelvic tilt. The CP patient often has an exaggerated neck curve and hypertonic extensor muscles in the lower back.

How then, can a prism used with hyperopes, produce the kinds of change that we see in the CP patient? There are a couple of different hypotheses that I have come up with, one of which I feel is the best explanation for the improved motor control. I will use a case study at the end of the paper to show how I drew my conclusion.

The first hypothesis related to the lack of co-contraction of the flexor and extensor muscles in the CP patient. Often the stereotyped pattern, exhibited by the CP patient, shows an extensor pattern with little extensor control and little or no flexion in the trunk to counteract the extensors. My initial feeling regarding the base-down prism was that they worked through the flexors to allow a more normal co-contraction. However, there are a couple of reasons why this doesn't comfortably resolve how the prism works. One reason has to do with the fact that the reaction to base-down prism is to look up. Looking up is a movement made through extension. For the person with CP, this movement goes unopposed by a counterthrust involving the flexors. Lack of a counterthrust is of obvious disadvantage to having the prisms work since the whole premise on which their function is based is that of the counter-shift or counterbalance to ultimately shift the center of gravity from behind the person to within the body.

The other reason why this first hypothesis is unable to explain the advantageous response to base-down prism relates to the inordinate amount of flexion that would be needed to act as a counterbalance to the excessive extensor pull. In an intact neurological system, it is possible to see how flexor control would balance out the normally graded extensor movements. In the person with CP, the flexor control would have to go through tremendous fluctuations in order to maintain a balance with the extensor oscillations. Because these shifts from extension to flexion and back to extension are not seen clinically with the application of base-down prism, I feel that some other mechanism is operating.

The second hypothesis is tied in with the improved extension that is totally observable upon introduction of the base-down prism. The prism allows the CP patient to perform as if a neurological monitor were acting within the system to control the spikes in the neurological signals. This gating phenomenon reminded me of the gating mechanism that neuro-biologist, Steven Cool, Ph.D., refers to the area of the locus coeruleus located within the reticular formation.

The reticular formation, as a whole, seems to, "perform some kind of summation of the over-all nervous activity of the organism."

"Reticular influences on the muscles are…varied…the general muscle tone of the body – the degree of contraction that characterizes the normal resting muscles – is controlled by the reticular activating system. Interference with certain of the communication channels from the reticular system to the muscles, results in extreme muscular contraction: interference with other fibers of the reticular formation causes the muscles to relax completely. Electric stimulation or lesions in another part of the reticular activating system interfere with the normal dynamic balance of the body's servomechanisms in such a way as to cause rhythmic muscular quivering similar to the shaking palsy of Parkinson's disease," or the ballistic movements of cerebral palsy.

Generally, the locus coeruleus has been studied in relationship to the processing of visual information. Research points to its having a facilitating effect on visual processing. Researchers such as Kasamatsu and Pettigrew in 1979, Kasamatsu et al. in 1983, and Pettigrew in 1978, have stated that the locus coeruleus is involved with brain plasticity and what they term critical periods. The interesting point these investigators make is that with stimulation of the locus coeruleus, there seems to be no critical period. This area of the reticular formation acts as a gate for letting new visual information processing take place. Specifically, the locus coeruleus appears to determine what and how much sensory signal will get through, according to Cool in 1984.

The most striking part, to me, of the locus coeruleus research is its possible relationship to the CP patient and our use of base-down prism. The thinking amongst many scientists is that in a couple of forms of cerebral palsy the sensory system is a major contributor to the ungraded or ballistic types of movement seen in CP. Movement is very hard to control when the sensory feedback is not there to signal the person where they are in space or when they have reached the endpoint of a movement. When we use base-down prism on the CP patient, we may very well be working via the locus coeruleus to better control the fluctuations in muscle tone and allow graded movement to emerge. This may explain why there is controlled extension that is seen clinically on application of base-down prism with the CP patient.

Case Study

The patient was an adult ambulatory, independent female diagnosed as having a mixed form of cerebral palsy involving athetosis and ataxia. She was originally referred in because of a visual dysfunction. As is often found among the different forms of cerebral palsy, this patient was strabismic and anisometropic. She came into visual training and was able to develop some binocularity. However, the underlying motor dysfunction was restricting further visual development so the patient was put on a vacation from training and referred out to a neuro-developmental/Bobath trained physical therapist.

Postural appearance of the patient on entering the neuro-developmental therapy was the following as noted by the physical therapist: hips in flexion, with external rotation and abduction of the right leg, and internal rotation and adduction of the left leg. The shoulders were elevated, arms externally rotated, and the scapulae were widely abducted there was hyper-tonicity of the extensors and a lack of any flexor control. Head control was poor in all positions, and most noticeably absent in prone and supine. The existing head control in an upright position was mainly through a compensatory extensor pattern with hyperextension of the neck.

Early on in treatment, base-down prism was used to try to facilitate the treatment process. The results at that time were disappointing at best. The prism use was discontinued because there had been no change over a 3-4 month period. Once and only once the prisms were removed did the true depth of the compensatory pattern become apparent. A period of 1½ years passed before there was a significant reduction of the compensatory patterns. As the influence of the compensatory patterns diminished and was no longer dominating the movement patterns and postural set, it became possible to guide the emergence of more normal movement patterns. At this point we reintroduced the base-down prism. The amount of prism used was determined by observing the extent of righting reactions with varying degrees of prism.

Current clinical observations are the following: Without the base-down prism on, the patient's typical seated posture is with the head forward, the neck hyper-extended, shoulders elevated, arms forward, trunk rounded, and legs widely abducted to provide a wide and therefore stable base of support.

With the prism on and the patient seated, within approximately 10 seconds, there was the emergence of controlled extension in the trunk. The extension started in the lumbar region and spread upward to allow the head to come into balance with the body. The shoulders were normally depressed, and arms rested at the sides. With the improved trunk support there was no longer a need to keep the legs widely abducted. One of the most noticeable changes was in breathing. Usually, breathing was only from the upper chest and shoulder region.

With prism on, the breathing was controlled respiration starting abdominally and spreading throughout the chest.

The subjective responses of the patient to the prism use in sitting were: "I have more sense of support at the mid-back region...I don't feel the need to look down to keep from flying backward...and breathing seems much easier."

Observations of seating weight-shifting activities, anterior to posterior and lateral weight shifting: the usual responses are a brief maintenance of balance through small arcs of slow movements. With prism on, balance was maintained through extreme arcs of movement and rapid reversals of direction. At this point the appropriate righting and equilibrium responses emerged.

SUMMATION
In summation, I hope that our thoughts and observations will be of help to those of you who are or will be working with cerebral palsied patients. Both the physical therapist and I have seen the powerful effects of prism. Prism can have tremendous value in the treatment of the patient with cerebral palsy. However we would like to add a note of caution. When optometrists use base-down prism to modify vision, posture, and movement without the movement guidance of a patient with a neuro-developmental problem we may just be embedding a different and as inappropriate a pattern as the CP patient had prior to prism use.

Notes
Woolridge DE. The Machinery of the Brain. New York: McGraw-Hill, 1962: 67-69.
Kasamatsu, Pettigrew JD. preservation of binocularity after monocular deprivation in the striate cortex of kittens treated with 6-Hydroxydopamine. J Comp Neurol 1975;185: 139-162.
Kasamatsu et al. Restoration of neuronal plasticity in cat visual cortex by electrical stimulation of the locus coeruleus. Society Neurosci Abstracts 1983:9(2):911.
Pettigrew JD. The locus coeruleus and cortical plasticity. Trends in Neurosci 1978;1:73-74.
Cool SJ. The scientific basis for the functional/behavioral approach to vision care: A suggested physiological model for the role of attention and stress in the functional/behavioral approach to vision care.

Bibliography
Bobath B, Bobath, K. Motor Development in the Different Types of Cerebral Palsy. London, William Heinemann Medical Books Limited, 1975.

Fiorentino MR. A Basis for Sensorimotor Development – Normal and Abnormal; The influence of Primitive, Postural Reflexes on the Development and Distribution of Tone. Springfield, Charles C. Thomas, 1981.
Keats S. Cerebral Palso. Springfield, Charles C. Thomas, 1965.
Knott M, Voss DE. Proprioceptive Neuromuscular Facilitation. New York: Harper & Row, 1968.
Kraskin RA. Lens power in action. Santa Ana, CA: Optometric Extension Program Foundation Papers, Volume 54, Series 1, 9,12, 1982.
Luttgen K, Wells KF. Kinesiology. New York: Saunders College, 1982.

Eye Movements, Information Theory, and the Rules of Language

Ron Berger, O.D.
Columbia, MD

In the course of examining eye movements during the act of reading, one cannot help but notice the variability of movements of one person compared with others, the consistency of movements of one individual repeatedly tested on material of consistent grade level, and the variability of movements of the same individual on material of differing degrees of difficulty. Each individual appears to have developed a particular pattern of gathering symbolic information, a pattern that may very with different print styles and level of difficulty, but one that is reliably reproduced when there is no variation of print type or change in the degree of difficulty of reading material

Of great interest in a study such as this is that there are a number of individuals whose ocular movement patterns during the act of reading are excellent (i.e., a proper number of fixations and regressions are recorded) but whose comprehension is measurably below normal; conversely, there are also a number of individuals whose ocular movement patterns are very poor but whose comprehension level is consistently well above the expected values. As optometrists we are interested not only in developing smoother and more accurate ocular movement patterns, but also in exploring why some people develop reliable movements on their own and why some others do not.

Since we assume that a major endeavor of the visual system is the gathering of information, a search for such answers might begin with a study of what information is. As a scientific concept, information theory began with electronic communications, at the beginning of the twentieth century. In its pure form, information theory was first elucidated in two papers, published in 1948, by Claude Shannon, an engineer with Bell Telephone Laboratories. The papers consist of a set of mathematical theorems dealing with the problem of sending messages from one place to another quickly, economically, and efficiently.

Shannon's theorems start with the concept that information is so logical and precise that it can be placed into a formal framework of ideas. The theory of information is thus universal to the point that it holds true for any kind of information, for any system in which a message is relayed from one place to another. Shannon's expression for the amount of information, the first precise, scientific measure, was of the same form as the entropy principle, a mathematical expression of the tendency for all things to become less orderly when left to themselves. In the language of chemistry, entropy is the process by which energy, in the natural course of events, undergoes transformations to become less organized and thus less useful, degrading in quality but unchanged in quantity. Shannon's equations linked energy and information together, their connective element, entropy. While scientists in the early 1940s were working on the mathematics of communication with a problem-by-problem approach, Shannon now coherently described the parameters of the science of information theory.

Another individual who contributed to the science of information was Norbert Wiener. He was the founder of cybernetics, the science of maintaining order within a system. Entropy is the tendency for all things to become disorderly, and the random deviations from order are continually corrected by the mechanism of cybernetics, which may be thought of as a regulatory mechanism, which enforces consistency according to the laws of any given system. Natural selection can be described as a cybernetic system in that it disallows genetic mutations, which deviate from the norm in undesirable ways.

Wiener was given the job of helping Bell Laboratories to improve the success of anti-aircraft fire against German bombers in World War II. They needed automatic devices to track an aircraft, compute its position, direction, and speed, and most critically, predict where it would be by the time the anti-aircraft shell reached the target area. Until this time, gun crews were essentially gambling, since they were relying on radar signals that were distorted by random electrical atmospheric interference. In addition, they were confronted with German pilots who certainly were doing their best to not be predictable. The imperfect state of radar technology presented Wiener with the task of separating the orderly message (where the plane was going) from the disorder of the unwanted electrical interference, or noise. In communication parlance, noise is anything that corrupts the integrity of a message. The weaker the signal from the plane, the more it is contaminated by random atmospheric noise obtained by the radar receiver circuits. He also realized that the sending of messages, the project that Shannon was working on at the same time, had a great deal in common with Brownian motion, the link being statistics, a branch of the theory of probability.

Now, a message is defined as a sequence of events spread out over time, events that are not known in advance. In mathematical terms a series of events like that is called "stochastic," from the Greek term *stochos*, to guess. The series are not totally unpredictable, but they do contain elements of the unknown. While you cannot say for sure what the price of a given share of stock will be in two days, you can make an educated guess. In the same way, a sentence in English is a series of letters and words obeying certain statistical rules. It is internally consistent, so that if a person knows the rules of the language, the sequence is not completely unpredictable. Given the first half of the sentence, you may be able to guess the second half, or be able to predict part of it. The point of a message, however, the reason for writing it, is that something new or unexpected should result; otherwise, there would be no reason to write the sentence at all.

Predictions involve the probable track of a grain in water, the probable fluctuation in the price of a share of stock, the probable arrangement of letters and words on a page. The mathematician, in making a prediction, considers not one future, but a multiplicity of futures. Statistics deals not with any single piece of data, but with a pattern of many possible events, each with a certain likelihood of being realized.

Weiner found that predicting where a plane will be several seconds from now is a problem for statistics to solve. The probable path of the plane is treated as one of many possible paths, and the problem of separating aircraft signals from noise is accomplished, likewise, statistically. Messages display a certain pattern, and the pattern will change in a manner determined partly by its past history. A single item of information, like a signal or a letter or a radar blip, makes no sense. Information is conveyed only when something is transmitted that changes the listener's knowledge. The listener is in a state of uncertainty as to what message he will hear, but he will know that is will be one of a range of possible messages, i.e., it will exist within a context. It will not be impossible to decipher or it would not be called information. The listener's mind will contain a number of possible actualities, thus excluding the other possibilities and resolving the listener's uncertainty. A greater amount of uncertainty is resolved if the message chosen is one of a large number of possibilities and if it is one of the more unlikely of those possibilities. An actual message must be considered not in isolation (like a single radar blip), but in relation to all possible messages, just as the actual path of a plane is part of a pattern that includes other possible paths. This is a point of central importance in information theory, that no signal is considered in isolation. Wiener was quite successful in his methodology, for the success rate in destroying enemy bombers rose from 10% to over 50% after his system went into effect.

Shannon's project, during the same time Wiener was dealing with separating signals from noise for Bell Labs, involved sending and deciphering secret codes. It was this work which enabled him to clarify his new theory of information, in particular suggesting how to separate messages from noise, or order from disorder, in a communication system. He started with the assumption that humans possess the most complex communication network on earth, and that human language is a code, one that preserves the orderly structure of messages of speech. Noise adds to and distorts messages, thereby rendering them less reliable; there must be a way of reducing noise so that symbol sequences sent by a source reach their destination unimpaired.

Shannon found that in nearly all forms of communication, more messages are sent than are truly necessary to convey information. Such additional messages diminish unexpectedness, the surprise effect, of the information itself, making it more predictable. This extra ration of predictability is redundancy, and it is an extremely important concept in information theory. Redundancy acts as a constraint, limiting entropy or reducing the number of ways in which the parts of the system can be arranged.

A message conveys no information unless some prior uncertainty exists about what the message will contain. The greater the uncertainty, the larger the amount of information the person will get when the uncertainty is resolved. There is a profound relationship between information and probability. When a roulette wheel is spun, total uncertainty exists until the ball comes to rest, at which time all uncertainty is resolved and becomes information. A page of English also creates and resolves uncertainty, but the uncertainty is not the same as in games of chance. While the roulette player cannot predict the outcome of a spinning wheel, a reader is not in such a poor state, for he may very well be able to predict the next letters or words in a sentence, on the basis of what he has already seen. The reason for this is that language, unlike coins or roulette wheels, is not a system in which all outcomes are neither equally possible nor equally predictable.

A written message is never completely unpredictable, for then it would be only nonsense, only noise. To be understandable, to convey meaning, it must conform to rules of spatial structure, sensibility, and spelling; these rules, known to the writer and the reader in advance, reduces uncertainty. They make the message partially predictable. Rules are a form of redundancy, and they are responsible for making the message of language different from the messages of a roulette wheel. Roulette messages are all equally probable, but the rules of language make certain letters and groups of letters, and certain sequences of words, more probably than others, and therefore more predictable.

In English, as in all languages, redundancy is of more than one kind. One type of redundancy consists of the rules of spelling, the effect of which is that certain letters appear more often than other letters over a fairly long stretch of text. The letter "E" for example, appears more than three times as often as it would if sentences were constructed by stringing letters together at random. This unequal probability in the average use of letters are recognized by Samuel Morse when he devised his code using the shortest sequence of dots and dashes for the most commonly used letters of the alphabet. The E, of course, received the briefest representation, a single dot.

A second type of redundancy arises from the fact that the probability of a certain letter occurring in a word depends, to some extent, on the letters that precede it. An example of one such rule is "I" before "E" except after "C." Oftentimes it is very easy to predict letters following a given sequence, i.e., the letter following "th" is very likely, although not absolutely certain, to be a vowel. The probability approaches certainty that the letter following a "q" will be a "u."

Shannon tried a number of ways to estimate the amount of redundancy in English text. He used his knowledge of secret codes to compress passages of prose into their common denominators, much as one would do to place a classified ad. He would play games such as opening a book and announcing the first letter of a sentence, then ask an individual to guess the next letter, over and over until the sentence was correctly completed. Each wrong guess would result in the correct letter being given. For example:

```
THE  ROOM  WAS  NOT  VERY  LIGHT  A  SMALL  OBLONG
___   ROO_  ___  NOT  V___  _I___  _  SM___  OB____

READING  LAMP  ON   THE  DESK  SHED   GLOW  ON
REA____  ____  O_   ___  D___  SHED   GLO_  O_

POLISHED  WOOD  BUT  LESS  ON  THE  SHABBY  RED  CARPET
P_L_S___  _O__  BU_  L_S_  O_  ___  SH____  RE_  C_____
```

Of the 103 letters in the sentence, the player needed 48, from which the sentence was correctly predicted. From the player's point of view, 63 of the letters were redundant, because they were predictable given a knowledge of the rules of spelling, structure, and sense.

Shannon concluded from his work that given a sample of eight letters, English is 50% redundant. For sequences of up to 100 letters, redundancy rises to almost 75%. It is even higher for whole pages or chapters, where the reader has the opportunity to familiarize himself with the statistics of the text, including its theme and literary style.

Redundancy reduces error by making certain letters and groups of letters more probable, increasing predictability. Words contain more letters than are strictly necessary for understanding, and sentences contain more words than are necessary. Redundancy also makes complexity possible. The more complex a system, the more likely one of its parts will malfunction. Redundancy is a means of keeping a system running in the presence of malfunction, a means of providing comprehension of a text even when a percentage of words are unreadable or incomprehensible.

When Shannon statistically analyzed language, he chose as his unit of information the binary digit or "bit," and defined it as a simple choice between two equally probable messages. It is a "yes" or "no" response to the hypothetical question: "Is it this one?" Either answer resolves all uncertainty in the mind of the person receiving the message, because he knows which of the two possible messages is the actual one. This type of code needs only two symbols, "1" for "yes" and "0" for "no." This code is adequate for any question whose answer is one of two possibilities.

If there are more than two possibilities from which to choose, more bits will be needed to resolve the uncertainty, Suppose on the roulette wheel that there are four alternatives; red and even, black and even, red and odd, or black and odd. The uncertainty must be measured by two binary digits rather then one, since two questions must be asked. The first question is "Is it either red and even or black and even?" If the answer is "0" or "no," the next question is "Is it red and odd?" The answer "1," or "0" resolves all uncertainty. Doubling the number of possible messages increases the uncertainty by one question to which there is a "yes" or "no" answer, or by one bit.

This procedure is less simple when all the possibilities are not equally probable, and when the system contains some redundancy. Certain letters or clusters of letters that are seen infrequently require a larger number of bits to decode them. The pair of letters "th," seen frequently, can be coded into just two bits, while a seldom used pair like "lc" would require 16 bits. Coding the entire English language is virtually impossible, but the human brain does a considerably adequate job.

Dr. William Bennett, Jr., of Yale's School of Engineering, used computers to translate statistical rules into language. He used Shakespeare's plays as his statistical language model, and calculated that a trillion monkeys typing on a typewriter at the rate of ten keys per second would take over a trillion years to produce the sentence, "To be or not to be; That is the question." However, as he applied simple rules of probability, his time line changed radically.

The first program change went from equal probabilities for each letter to an arrangement in which certain letters appeared more frequently than others, just as they do in the play Hamlet. The four most common letters were "e," "o," "t," and "a," the least common, "j," "x," "q," and "z." With these new instructions, the computer monkeys still produced gibberish, but now it had some hint of structure:

NCRDEERH HMFIOMRETW OVRLA OSRIE IEOBUTOGIM NUD SEEWU

The second stage of programming concerned which letters are most likely to appear at the beginning and end of words, and which pairs of letters ("th," "he," "ue," and "ex") are used most often. The monkey's result this time was:

ANED AVECA AMEREND TIN NF MEP FOR'T SESILORK
TITIPOFELON HERIOSHIT MY ACT

During the second stage of programming, an inordinately large number of indelicate words and expletives appeared. Bennett suspects that one-syllable obscenities are among the most probable sequences of letters used in normal language. From a statistical standpoint, swearing thus has low information content. When Bennett programmed the computer to take into account triplets of letters, where the probability of one letter is affect by the presence of the two letters before it, half the words were correct English words. At the fourth level of programming, groups of four letters were considered, and the results were 90% correct words. One such computer run came up with:

TO DEA NOW NAT TO BE WILL AND THEM BE DOES SOESORNS CALAWROUTOULD

Given statistically correct rules of language, it appears that a computer monkey could write classical prose.

As Bennett proceeded through his four levels of programming, adding more and more redundancy, the produced tests acquired more and more structure, or became easier to predict. Dr. Lila Gatlin, working on biological aspects of information theory, pointed out two different kinds of redundancy, and applied them to Bennett's computer work. The first kind of redundancy is the statistical rule that some letters are more likely to appear more often than others in a passage of text. This is called context-free redundancy and measures the extent to which a sequence of symbols generated by a message source departs from the completely random state in which each symbol is just as likely to appear as any other symbol. The second kind of redundancy is called context-free redundancy, and measures the extent to which the individual symbols have departed from a state of perfect independence from one another, departed from a state in which context does not exist.

Increasing context-free redundancy is a safeguard against error, because it makes sequences more predictable. If a page has more "x's" and "z's" than "e's," we know something is wrong, for the rules of statistical structure will have been violated. On the other hand, context-free redundancy is also expensive, meaning that it can place severe limits of the variety of messages that can be sent. If you could only use certain letters over and over again, the number of words you could make would be severely curtailed.

Context-sensitive redundancy also makes sequences of symbols more predictable, by setting up relationships between letters. Yet context-sensitive redundancy is not as expensive, for it does not restrict messages to only a few letters. It permits greater variety, while at the same time controlling errors. English is higher in context-sensitive than in context-free redundancy, thus allowing for the rich variety in language. It can always communicate new ideas, but only within the framework of familiar rules of structure and sense.

The modern theory of language bears a striking resemblance to the statistically oriented theory of information. Noam Chomsky, the foremost thinker of language theory, pays a great deal of attention to order, regularity, and form in language. He concentrates on syntax, and on redundancy, the entropy-reducing elements in an information system that separates messages from noise. Like Shannon, he concentrates on message systems as a whole rather than with single messages and with the common qualities of the message source and the message receiver. He regards language as a well-defined system on the basis of form, and spoken and written language are understandable to the reader because the reader is aware of the same coding principles as the writer or speaker. This allows "noise," in the form of mistakes, slips, of the tongue, repetitions, distractions, misprints, and syntactical or grammatical errors to be eliminated or restructured by the listener or reader, so that the meaning of the message is transmitted despite noise in the system. Chomsky considers that a universal grammar exists, one that reduces improbability and makes communication of messages not only possible but also highly likely.

Chomsky's theory of language is based on a series of rules that conform to the laws of statistics and probability, much as Shannon's laws defining the theory of information. They provide for an endless variety of language combinations, but most importantly provide for communication based on knowledge of rules by both the message source and the message receiver. They are inundated by redundancy, context-free and context-sensitive, that both sets rules and provides for complexity that constrains the usage of the language parts while allowing for creativity and surprise.

The relationship of eye movements to these principles is certainly not a totally clear one, but placing eye movements into the context of information theory and language theory can be helpful. Some of the consistency that we see in the eye movements of good readers become more understandable, some of the variability of eye movements from person to person become more understandable; the ability of one person with very poor eye movements to extract a high degree of comprehension out of some reading material becomes explainable, and the inability of some children to learn how to read well despite the availability of accurate eye movements becomes better understood and thus easier to remediate.

When approached from a statistical viewpoint, incorporating the theories of information and language, eye movements during the course of reading (and all eye movements) become responses to the probability that uncertainty will be resolved. The movements become barometers by which we can measure how well an individual has learned the rules of language, and how well an individual can reduce the number of possible alternatives in a given section of print he has not yet seen, to the most probable likelihoods by the process of visualization.

Observations on Characteristics of Distance Blur

Gregory Kitchener, O.D.
Cincinnati, OH

Dr. Elliot Forrest presented a paper at last year's Symposium entitled, "Visual Imagery and the Plateau Spiral in Myopia Control." In that paper he made several interesting points about his own approach to optometry and included the observations of one particular patient. I would like to elaborate and continue on the track, which Dr. Forrest started with some comments and observations from my own experience.

Dr. Forrest stated that he was a proponent of a philosophical approach, which favored, "the view that, for the most part, we are active participants in the selective adaptive outcomes (such as myopia) that so many of us wind up with." He goes on to say that in therapy we must have the patient "begin to experience that the ability to change and improve their status also rests with themselves."

Dr. Forrest then related an anecdote, which described his use of the Plateau Spiral with a myopic patient. The patient described a "circular gray disc" that prevented him from seeing the distal end of the spiral, which he was visualizing. The patient commented, "Then as I thought about it, I began to recognize that since I was the one who was visualizing and creating the spiral in my mind, I must also be the one who was creating the gray disc that was blocking my vision." Later he states, "It seems that although I vehemently dislike being nearsighted, at some deeper level I must want to be nearsighted otherwise I would not be setting up any blocks. Some part of me obviously does not want to deal with things off in the distance."

Throughout the discussion between Dr. Forrest and his patient, myopia is discussed as a negative, i.e. a problem. I would like to return to Dr. Forrest's tenet, "We are active participants in the selective adaptive outcomes (such as myopia)..." and add an opinion that behavior is purposeful and logical. This establishes a framework for observation in which the individual is required to make decisions based on limited information. Through active processes, he chooses those solutions that seem most adequate for meeting his needs as he sees them. I think that it is then possible to look at both sides of the coin simultaneously, and view myopia as both a solution and a problem. I see this as the basis of a holistic approach.

Dr. Forrest stated, "It is only as more appropriate questions begin to be asked that more revealing responses surface and often it only takes one insightful patient or one insightful interaction to open the door to new perspectives." I would approach this slightly differently by adding that if we open up our testing situations so that patients can show us and tell us what they see, and if we can become sensitive enough to see what they are doing, then insightful patients and insightful interactions are plentiful.

One test that I find useful in this type of investigation is a distance stereo test, which I use routinely at the completion of the analytical examination. Dr. Bruce Wolff, who has used it for many years, first introduced me to this procedure. Based on his clinical experience, the test is used in the examination sequence at the s.a. Noel Center. A 2x2 stereo Vectographic slide is projected onto the screen at the end of the examination room. Stereo Optical Company originally produced the slide. It has been reproduced and is available through the s.a. Noel Center. A grid approximately six feet wide by four feet high consists of five rows of the numbers one through six. Each row is labeled on the left side with a letter from "A" at the top to "E" at the bottom. The numbered elements have a variety of crossed, uncrossed, and zero disparities. The patient wears a pair of Polaroid analyzers. When fully resolved, the elements occupy a very large visual volume. Indeed the testing is designed to examine the quality of this stereo volume rather than obtaining the more conventional stereo acuity measurement. As you might assume, all elements, regardless of disparity, are focused on the screen.

The testing is started, rather simply, by asking the patient what he sees. Patients exhibit many interesting approaches to this visual problem and their specific observations and language are clinically useful and often fascinating. One observation that startled me initially has recurred with surprising frequency. Patients will report that some of the elements are blurred. Occasionally they will report this as differences in contrast. I find it interesting that similar figures on the same chart will be blurred and clear simultaneously. The stereo-localization of the blurred elements is typically distorted. The blurred elements all seem to have the same type of disparity and most frequently this is uncrossed disparity. These are the elements that should appear beyond the plane of the screen. If the patient begins to report a more canonical stereo-localization, the blur will no longer be apparent. Patients often seem unaware of the change from blurred to clear.

Blur is traditionally considered to be a product of the refractive components of the ocular apparatus. Even in translation to more behavioral terms, blur is associated with the Identification aspects of vision. The blur associated with testing in the analytical examination generally affects all elements in the field uniformly. In crossed-cylinder testing only a portion of the field is affected, but this is usually consistent with and predictable from the optics of the cylindrical lens. The shifts in blur during crossed-cylinder testing are associated with the posturing of Identification. The blur that I have described affects only specific, widely scattered elements of a static field. The only common factor I have found is the distorted stereo-localization. This seems to be a type of binocular blur that is more closely related to the Centering aspects of vision.

I have seen this type of response frequently (but not exclusively) in the early stages of myopia adaptation. I have begun to see this as a part of many complaints of distance blur. This is especially true when they are accompanied by orientation difficulties such as problems with night driving. A true integration of Centering and Identification factors in the development of and the resolution of distance blur could be more compatible with a holistic approach. Approaches based on a limited view of vision, with an emphasis on refractive and accommodative factors, may not be sufficient to explain the distance blur which patients perceive. Even Identification and Centering are insufficient if the processes are viewed sequentially. I have already pointed out that, viewed holistically, myopia can be seen as both a solution and a problem simultaneously. From this viewpoint I begin to see that there might be negative aspects to a "successful" therapy aimed at the restoration of normal distance acuity. In conclusion, I would like to remember Dr. Elliot Forrest and his many contributions, and encourage each of us to follow his lead in seeking "new perspectives" through "more appropriate questions."

The Gesellian Contributions and Their Impact Upon Our Optometric Heritage

G. N. Getman, O.D., D.O.S., Sc.D.
Waldorf, MD

Exactly 50 years ago this coming Thursday – January 29th, I was issued a piece of paper stating that I had earned the title DOCTOR OF OPTOMETRY. If the elapse of so many years did not give me the prerogative for some reminiscing, I would still take the privileges of personal experiences and participations to speak to the subject assigned me by Dr. Kraskin. In this process, I am finding it most difficult to dwell entirely upon only one of the five most significant events of the past 45 years (and the individuals involved) when all five have brought us to the possibility of a most enviable position among all clinical disciplines. Further, all of these five have been so closely inter-related and symbiotic it is impossible to isolate one of these five for insular discussion. However, the time limits demand this be attempted, and I will just briefly mention the five and then concentrate on the one that my personal bias insists is the most significant of the five.

In chronological order these are: The Baltimore Myopia Project that taught optometry the immeasurable differences between classical othoptics and optometric visual training, and brought us the realization that the only "magic" factor was the patient's desire to improve his, or her, visual abilities above and beyond the special designs of our instrumentation. (Parenthetically, I must comment that some of today's entrepreneurs have not yet learned this fact.) The second event was the Original Yale Clinic of Child Development and the very spacious influences of Dr. Arnold Gesell and his devoted staff. This is the one of the five I will be more fully describing momentarily. Third was the Ohio State Summer Classes under the impact of Professor Samuel Renshaw, where we did to each other what we dared not to do to our patients. Our zeal to reach greater understandings of the visual system and its processes of performance resulted in visual conditions some of the participants never fully remedied in the years that followed. Fourth, was the multidimensional influence of Dr. Darrell Boyd Harmon, and his concepts of the totality of the physiopsychological relevancies which influenced – and were influenced by – vision. These were actually the primary concepts analyzed and catalyzed by A.M. Skeffington so we could come to the point of describing our profession as a behavioral clinical entity. And, finally, the fifth of these events was the Glen Haven Colorado Achievement Camp where optometry tested and proved its convictions that visual training – *a la* Gesell, Renshaw, Harmon and Skeffington – could bring intellectual and behavioral changes in damaged children that no other clinical profession had ever considered or even attempted. At this time I cannot avoid commenting that what we learned from the Gesellian environment brought both body and soul to all of the other four situations and events that would have not been present if the Yale Clinic of Child Development had not been available to us.

From a completely personal perspective – I am repeatedly awestruck with the fact that I had such extensive opportunities for such intimate participations in all five of these situations. As of this moment, I am now the only person still around who can make such a statement, and I know I am the only person who can look back on each of these with a wealth of primary memories that allow me the prerogative to attempt an account of some parts of the entire story of the evolution of developmental and behavioral optometry. I deeply appreciate the invitation from Bob Kraskin to present a portion of the story here this noon.

Actually, this account must start back in the early 1930s when Dr. Arnold Gesell needed a stenographer skilled enough in shorthand to collect all of his comments and observations on the children he was examining. Miss Glenna Bullis came out of the local business college course for this position, and in a very short time Gesell found the transcriptions contained pertinent and valuable details he had not directly dictated. It became obvious that Miss Bullis was a very keen and insightful observer of children's behavior and had simply added her observations in her desire to be of greater service to Dr. Gesell. In our numerous very personal conversations over the years in which I participated in the Clinic program Gesell frequently commented to me that Miss Bullis had been the most valuable addition ever made to the Clinic staff.

Miss Bullis had a nephew who was having unexplained difficulties in school – especially in reading classes. Miss Bullis found a Keystone stereoscope and the usual DB visual skills cards put away on a closet shelf at the Clinic. She was determined to explore this instrument to see if it might provide some clues to the problems her nephew was experiencing. Dr. Vivian Ilg, an optometrist and sister of Dr. Francis Ilg, another pediatrician on the Clinic staff, encouraged Miss Bullis and gave what assistance she could. Miss Bullis called one of the New Haven optometrists to ask for help. As this acquaintance grew and prospered, the optometrist suggested Miss Bullis attend a seminar being presented by Dr. A.M. Skeffington. This opened another acquaintance that eventually led to Miss Bullis's regular attendance at the St. Louis Visual Training conference where she immediately caught the attention of all present with her insights on visual development and her probing questions about visual behavior as it related to the learning process in children. I was completely entranced with Miss Bullis and her suggestions about vision and learning since I was already deeply involved in the visual problems of children.

This friendship between us grew to include her many visits to our Minnesota home, and a constant stream of communications about children and their visual abilities, I was serving my two weeks on the optometric staff at the Baltimore Myopia Project when Arnold Gesell – at Miss Bullis's urging – came by to see what was being done there. World War II troop movement had cancelled my train reservations and kept me in Baltimore an extra day – the day Gesell came to visit. The rooms occupied by this seminal visual training project, the number of children being trained, and the number of staff at work there prevented our spending much time in these crowded rooms. As a result, Gesell and Getman spent a greater part of the day seated on the floor out in the corridor just outside the project space. I have frequently remarked that I am undoubtedly the only person alive who ever saw Arnold Gesell sitting on the floor deep in clinical discussion with another adult. In these very special moments of philosophical exchange Gesell emphatically expressed his confidence that the Clinic of Child Development had pretty well concluded their studies of infant and young child development, and had all significant benchmarks of early human development identified. However, he said: (and I repeat his comments verbatim from vivid memory) "We have closed all conceptual doors except the one on vision – we still know very little about this completely unique human ability because we can get no help from the Department of Ophthalmology in the Yale Medical School." As the conversation continued and I was able to provide some scanty insights to visual performance in children far beyond anything obtained from other departments at Yale, Gesell asked me if I would be interested in coming to the Yale Clinic as a resource person – *IF* the finances could be found. Of course I expressed my interest and assured him I would check with my family and think it over.

I immediately discussed this with A.M. Skeffington who also expressed an interest in the possibilities it offered. At this time in the evolution of the Optometric Extension Program, both Skeffington and Dr. E.B. Alexander were enjoying a close personal relationship with the president of the American Optical Company (AO). This was a time when the American Optical Company WAS an optical company with serious ongoing research in human vision under the direction of Dr. Paul Boeder – a psychophsyiologist with a primary interest in human sight. Skeffington and Alexander had so impressed Walter Stewart, an AO president with the importance of low plus lenses that the AO Company was the only source of plus lenses of less than 1.00 diopter powers. Skeffington and Alexander went to Southbridge, Mass., the home of AO, and so influenced Stewart that he convinced his Board of Directors to underwrite the Yale Clinic of Child Development and its study of visual development. There are numerous reports of the actual dollar amount of this grant. I only know that in today's money values the sum provided by the AO Company would be in the hundreds of thousands of dollars. This sum was enough to maintain the entire staff and program of the Clinic and came at a time when Yale University was determined to enforce Gesell's retirement because of his contributions that were contradicting the pathological philosophies which were the "laws" of the medical profession at that time. The amount of money was significant enough that Gesell's retirement was delayed more than four years until the infant vision study was completed and the book, *Vision Its Development in Infant and Child*,[1] was completed and off the press in December of 1949. Fortunately, I had the privilege of being a part of the project from the start of the infant vision study until the book went to press in the spring of 1949.

There are many, many anecdotes that could be included here – all of which would give a fuller appreciation of this entire situation. These anecdotes would have to include the visits of Dr. George Crow of Los Angeles who came by three or four times a year especially while I was present – so we could carefully and cautiously go over the data we were gathering to be sure it was clinically consistent with what we already

---

[1] *Gesell A, Ilg FL, Bullis GE. Vision Its Development in Infant and Child. Optometric Extension Program Foundation, 1921 E. Carnegie Ave., Ste. 3-L, Santa Ana, CA 92705, (949) 250-8070.*

knew as optometric clinical fact. These visits by George Crow were spectacular in many ways. The Crow and Gesell personalities were as different as your imagination can possibly conjure; yet these two men established an interpersonal respect and communication beyond all description. It never came to a "George and Arnold" relationship but there was a distinct difference between the sounds of "Dr. Crow" and "Dr. Gesell" when they addressed each other. George insisted that his daily lunch had to be a glass of beer and a beef sandwich. The only place such was available was a dingy corner saloon where Gesell and Crow received the gifts of conversations that could not have happened anywhere else. The rest of the Clinic staff – especially Francis Ilg and Louise Bates (the staff psychologist) never did believe my accounts of these noontime sessions because they knew Gesell would never visit such a place, nor drink a glass of beer in such a place. Glenna Bullis, knowing Gesell better than any of the rest of the staff, and knowing George Crow from her visits to the visual training conferences, fully recognizing the mind-stretching that was coming out of the dingy saloon visits, and had many laughs over the situations that arose in the dingy corner beer joint.

The visits by Dr. Crow had numerous other results, and there is a multitude of anecdotes that could be told in this regard. We both stayed at the Taft Hotel while we were in New Haven and this gave us the opportunity to review each day's observations and to plan our activities for the next day. These evenings together, with Miss Bullis to give us the intimate guidance we needed to cope with the rest of the staff, had tremendous impact on everything I did while I was a part of the infant vision study. I could only afford to stay in New Haven for short periods of time – usually one week and no more than two weeks at a time. My family had to have food and shelter, and the office appointment schedule had to be kept if solvency was to be maintained. The stipend from the University, out of the AO grant, covered travel and hotel expenses but did not begin to cover the expense of being absent from the office. Thus, I had to make the New Haven trips according to the money available at home in addition to the AO grant. This turned out to be a tremendous blessing in disguise because each time I returned to my Minnesota practice; I applied and tested what I was learning at New Haven. If what we were contemplating at the Clinic did not hold with the children I saw in my office, or if what I thought was true of the Minnesota children was not holding for Connecticut youngsters, we had the immediate opportunity to review and re-evaluate. The scarcity of money actually gave us a wealth of information we could not have achieved had money been in unlimited supply.

It is completely impossible to pass this aspect of the total experience without taking a moment to give high praise to Arnold Gesell for his intellectual integrity, his open-mindedness and his willingness to listen and analyze what others from a very different frame of reference were telling him. He would repeatedly say: "We must go through that again," or "We must not overlook what we are saying now when we get farther into our study here." I had the privileges – privileges that goose-bump me to this day – of sitting across the desk from Gesell in the total privacy of his office while we would probe and scrutinize each conclusion we generated over what was being observed in the nursery, on the playground, or in Miss Bullis's office where I was doing the visual investigations. Gesell was truly a great man. In all of the years I knew him – and I still am confident I came to know him in a way and to an extent unequalled by any other person, with the exception of Miss Glenna Bullis – he never hindered nor doubted the thoughts of those around him. Nor did he ever look down upon another person as being unqualified or unworthy of his attention. His private office door was always open to me – no matter how insignificant my request of him. Unfortunately, not all of his staff was as sincere and intellectually honest, and there were some of the staff frictions that always exist in such a project as this exploration of totally virgin territory in the study of human infants and very young children.

There is one that will give you an even greater respect for this man. The book had finally reached the printer's galley stage. We worked long hours over certain pages but all of the galley proofs had not arrived from the printer when it was again time for me to return home. The morning I was to leave the galleys for chapters 9 and 10 arrived. Gesell suggested I take them with me to read and appraise. I would take an overnight train from New York to Chicago; spend a useful day in Chicago and then take an overnight train to Sioux Falls, South Dakota. These Pullman ambiences were a delight to a boy from the country. I started reading these proofs after dinner on the train out of New York and never was able to pull down the berth in my Pullman roomette. A sleepless night completely altered the day of shopping in Chicago and the night between Chicago and Sioux Falls was equally sleepless. These two chapters were not right. They did not fit what I knew was optometrically true, and I was terribly disturbed over them. How could I possibly tell Gesell these two chapters were unacceptable?

After hours of tussling with the problem, I finally called Dr. Gesell on the phone to tell him of my concerns, and to also tell him that I had written pages of notes about these two chapters. His immediate response was to ask me when I would be able to return to New Haven for more work on these chapters, and to assure me that if these two chapters made me that uncomfortable there was surely something wrong with them that we could rewrite. I fully expected to be told that what had been written was the way it was to be sent to press, and to recognize my inadequacies and ignorance. Instead, this great man welcomed me back to New Haven a short time later and we did completely rewrite these two chapters with primary attention to the pages of notes the two sleepless nights had produced. I have only known a handful of individuals with such depth of integrity and character in these past 50 years – and I have known dozens who would not have given a country boy even a moment's consideration in similar circumstances. One other "famous" man, to whom I sent a requested critique of a book he was writing, has not spoken to me again in the past 30 years. There are only three or four non-optometrists for whom I have the respect and admiration I still hold for Dr. Arnold Gesell.

There is still another aspect of this entire experience which must be carefully detailed here because of its never-ending influence upon what we now recognize as behavioral optometry. I went to New Haven the first time with the full confidence that I was THE optometrist who would completely educate the Clinic staff about vision, and about the contributions they could expect from my profession. I had been clinically involved with young children for almost five years, and had already reported some significant clinical details no other optometrist had observed. There was absolutely no doubt in my mind about my abilities, my spectacular clinical insights on the visual abilities of children, or what to do about the visual problems of preschool children. I knew I was already an expert in the routine optometric examination of children, and readily acclaimed my ability to complete the Skeffington Analytical Sequence on 4- or 5-year-old youngsters. I was fully ready for the Yale staff – I just hoped they were as ready for me as I was for them.

This egotistical ecstasy lasted less than a couple of hours after arrival at the Clinic. I was taken into the office of Miss Bullis and introduced to an 18-month-old child and asked to make an appraisal of her visual status. There was a phoropter of my choice beside the small examining chair, and this child would have absolutely nothing to do with any of such gadgetry. She also vehemently refused to allow me to get any closer than 2 or 3 feet, and turned her face into her mother's shoulder the moment I brought a trial lens into view. After all the cajoling and coaxing I could employ, I suddenly realized I knew absolutely nothing about conducting a visual examination on a reluctant, frightened 18-month-old child. All my egotism disappeared, and my gross incompetence was obvious to everyone gathered to see a spectacular optometric demonstration. I was suddenly face-to-face with how little I really knew and how inadequate I really was.

Fortunately, I had developed some skills in the use of the retinoscope. I had learned how to obtain refractive neutrality quickly and accurately. I had been fortunate to learn how to neutralize prescriptions with trial lenses as I spent high school time in my father's office. The morning after graduation I found myself in the lens surfacing department of an optical laboratory in Sioux City, Iowa, where the lab foreman so mistrusted the available lensometer that he also insisted all finished lenses be checked by hand neutralization. I became adept enough at this to confidently estimate lens powers within half diopters just by holding them up to an optical cross on the laboratory wall. As I sat in front of the 18-month-old child I suddenly also realized that I had a retinoscope and that retinoscopy would have to be accomplished without the use of any neutralizing lenses. I moved across the room and did all distance retinoscopy estimations from a distance of 15 feet from a position immediately below the line drawing pictures we used to attract the child's visual attention at far point. It was here that the changes in the brightness of the retinoscopic reflexes became so vividly apparent, and we were able to relate these reflex changes with the attention and interpretation attitudes of the child. Instead of merely judging the reflex brightness as a determinant of a dioptrics neutral (as all of us were taught to do in school) here came the recognition that the brightness changes could also occur without dioptrics variations and we were seeing a completely new aspect of refractive status and retinal sensitivity. Out of these first experiences of seeing the retinoscopic reflexes from an entirely new and different point of reference has come more than 40 years of appreciation of the retinoscope as the instrument which allows observations of cognitive and intellectual processes that range far beyond mere dioptrics values of a camera-like eye. This small child's refusal to cooperate with me opened a whole new concept of visual function, and has brought a wealth of clinical data no other discipline enjoys.

There is no doubt in my mind over the probability that this mid-40s "discovery" of the unrealized values the retinoscope has, had a greater impact upon our profession than any other single event in our clinical evolution. It is startling to find that the reflex color changes were beautifully described by Skeffington in his 1928 book, *Procedure in Ocular Examination.* Here, almost 60 years ago he wrote of the "oriflamme" or red reflex and the "argentums" or silvery reflex. Skeffington's 1931 book, *Differential Diagnosis in Ocular Examination*, really brings a reader up short when he states: "It may be a hard saying but nevertheless a truthful one that the refractionist is dealing not so much with the eye itself, but almost entirely with the brain." Eighteen years later Gesell wrote: "These speculations (about the explanation of the reflex changes) have little bearing on the value of the retinoscope as an investigatory or diagnostic instrument. It is enough to say that the evidence now available strongly indicates that the brightening and dulling of the retinal reflex are directly correlated with the activity of the higher nerve centers in the visual system...With the possibility of photo-electric instrumentation capable of making comprehensive records of retino-cortical responses, the retinoscope may take on added significance as a diagnostic device and as an aid in child-vision research." As recently as the January chapters from OEPF we find Dr. Mort Davis stating: "A retinoscope can tell the examiner more about the quality of the child's visual response than all of the drawings or motor behavior recordings combined." Taking these statements from the past 60 years, and a survey of the index to the OEPF chapters, where there are literally hundreds of pages of information on this single instrument, you might begin to recognize my bias and conviction that the retinoscope is the most important overpriced small flashlight ever manufactured. Perhaps one day in the not too distant future its values may be more widely recognized as a device which gives the behavioral optometrist insights completely unavailable to any other student of the human species.

If time and occasion allowed I could easily fill the rest of this day, and all of tomorrow, describing all that came about within one sector of optometry as a direct result of the time spent with Gesell and his staff at the original Clinic of Child Development. Its immediate influence was present in almost every project undertaken at the Ohio State summer classes after 1943. Project after project was designed to make further explorations of visual performance that could be observed and qualified through use of the retinoscope. The comparison of the retinal reflex changes with the tracings on the lie detector when a convict at the Ohio

State Prison was being interrogated were startling because the retinoscopic changes were consistently noted split seconds ahead of the lie detector's responses. The observations of the retinoscope changes present on adults brought new appreciations of the differences between acuity and recognition levels on visually demanding targets more than two miles away from the subject. An elaborate experimental arrangement provided the opportunity to clearly observe cognitive closure in subjects from an institution for the mentally retarded near the campus – mental processing that these subjects were supposedly unable to achieve according to standard psychological tests of intelligence. The retinoscopic observations of the influences of postural stress upon visual processing of critical information brought greater appreciation for the wealth of information Darrell Boyd Harmon was giving us. With these observations of body stresses while a gymnast was "practicing" his trampoline routines using visualization as a routine review procedure. In these two situations the Skeffington phrase "total organism" took on meaning for us the words alone could not possibly convey or communicate. In addition to all of these – so briefly and incompletely described here – were the realizations of the role that vision plays in the total learning process, and the midnight bull session experience with a highly regarded and top flight brain scientist when he served as a subject for the retinoscopic observations while this scientist was translating an English psychology text into Greek. Although there are still thousands of doubters – both inside and outside of optometry – this optometric understanding of the visual process via the retinoscope and its related optometric clinical procedures has made more positive contributions to thousands of students than can be justifiably claimed by any other discipline – including the education profession.

I truly regret that this is neither the time nor the place to regale you with hundreds of anecdotes that can be traced to the hours a couple of optometrists spent exploring the role of vision in human development under the tremendously insightful guidance and knowledge of Dr. Arnold Gesell and the intimate guidance of Miss Glenna Bullis. Many of these anecdotes are still hilariously amusing while others are still full of depressive heartbreak. The experiences and events which all came as a direct result of the Yale Clinic situation run the full spectrum of both fact and imagination. No matter how all of this might be interpreted and analyzed, no one will ever convince me that behavioral optometry would exist today if Glenna Bullis had not insisted Gesell visit the Baltimore Myopia Project, and gain his permission for her to attend optometric meetings; if Skeffington and Alexander had not been able to convince the American Optical Company to invest an immense sum of money in the work of Gesell and his staff; if I had not been forced to stay over an extra day in Baltimore so I could meet and visit Gesell, and if my beloved wife had not allowed me the freedom to spend weeks in Connecticut. As a result of those many, many absences I was never at home for any family emergency my very special wife, Clara, held the fort against all odds and family traumas. As I have so frequently stated from numerous platforms in these past 50 years, I have been the ultimate example of serendipity – of being in the right place at the right time doing the right things with the right people because of the love and support of a handful of special friends. I have only one regret – that each and every one of you could not have participated in this landmark event, and so many of its spin-offs, as I have. I shall be eternally grateful to a very gracious God for the years given me to see what has come out of those times we thought were unimportant and so insignificant while they were happening. All will have been completely worth every minute of it all if each of you will pick up your retinoscope during this coming week and look through it with new curiosities and awareness of what it can tell you about vision, its development and the behaviors directly resulting from the visual functions you can learn to observe. I know that many of you have only vaguely glimpsed the depth and breadth of vision and its role in human behavior. As I now complete my 50 optometric years, I can only offer you a simple challenge – do not allow yourself to sink into the imitations of those who know so much less about vision than you do, and who have none of the clinical potentials you possess. The visual development process which originates and structures all human behavior is the clinical arena that only the behavioral optometrist can occupy. As Skeffington repeatedly said to us over many years, this is the grail we can and must reach for and firmly grasp in our clinical uniqueness and professional devotions.

What is "The Core Philosophy?"

G. N. Getman, O.D., D.O.S., Sc.D.
Waldorf, MD

To an ancient Chinese philosopher goes the credit for saying, "If one wishes to deal accurately with something, one must first call it by its proper name." In a very recent speech by the World Affairs Council, Secretary of State, George P. Schultz said, "In ancient China, when familiar words and ways of thinking no longer accurately described the realities of the day, philosophers spoke of the need to 'rectify names' so that concepts would correspond to the new order of things."

In both of these instances lies the notion that the language one uses expresses the magnitude of the concepts one holds – and, at the same time – will influence the validity of the concepts one is developing. It is more and more apparent that there is a critical need in contemporary optometry to "rectify names" so our concepts will more properly correspond to the new order and advancements of our clinical philosophies.

In making such an effort, I would like to begin by attempting to "rectify" the language we use when we described what we have been calling BEHAVIORAL OPTOMETRY. I am especially eager to try such a venture because of the frequency of the use of this phrase – BEHAVIORAL OPTOMETRY – and its descriptions and discussions in terms that are more appropriate to the classical and traditional ways of thinking – those "ways of thinking that no longer accurately describe the realities of the day."

At least for my own comfort, I would describe BEHAVIORAL OPTOMETRY as: *the clinical study and appraisal of all those human behaviors that can be directly attributed to the processes of visual inspection, discrimination and interpretation of the surrounding lighted world, and its contents.* In choosing such a description, I am fully aware that there are mechanisms that can be observed and measured as parts of the basic functional system for visual performance. However, if we are to use the word behavioral as an adjective to describe a particular aspect of our professional activities then we must certainly look more carefully at the resulting actions of the individual than we do at the specifications of the contributing parts. If we are to continue to speak of vision as an emergent out of all the information processing systems, which influence it, the emerging behavior will be more important than the details of the mechanism. It is thus that the total is so much more than the sum of its parts, or the actions of *each* part.

However, in the same breath, and in the same instant, we must realize that there can be no behavior to observe if the parts are not making the contribution each is designed and coded to make. It is impossible to attend only to behavior without a degree of attention to its origins. It is this "horns of the dilemma" situation, which makes us clinicians instead of philosophers, and gives us the responsibility to work from the parts to behavior, and simultaneously from the behavior to the parts. Only this bi-directional thought and action by us can possibly bring the mediations we determine to be necessary for the benefits we offer our patients.

In the efforts to come to some conclusions in all of this, we repeatedly refer to what we call "THE CORE PHILOSOPHY." Almost as often as we refer to this central idea, upon which we base our clinical efforts, questions arise about it all. This has been especially true in the past few months when we optometrists gather to discuss our procedures, the results of our regimens, and the explanations/reasons/rationales we can offer. All of the specific reasons for the questions being raised need not be itemized here, but there must be some attempt to delineate THE CORE PHILOSOPHY before too much more time passes; mainly because there are now so many obvious misinterpretations and distractions impacting upon the basic concepts which underlie the clinical optometric philosophy passed down through the past 60 years from the unique contributions of A.M. Skeffington, and his associates.

One reason for the question: "What is the core philosophy?" comes out of the glibness, and the casualness, with which so many optometrists use this phrase either in discussion, or as background for lecture platform comments. I am emphatically reminded of one of our 15 grandchildren who is approaching the age of 5, and who has enjoyed two very successful years in a splendid nursery school environment. Recently, as we discussed his nursery school activities with him, Danny stated that the children salute the flag and say the Pledge of Allegiance each morning before they start their group playtime. Danny offered to say it for us, and proceeded to do so without the slightest hesitancy or mistake. After the applause died down, I asked him if he knew what this pledge meant, and why they repeated it each morning at school. He casually admitted that he did not know what it was all about, but offered the information that they said it because it was what they were supposed to say each morning. I could not avoid the thought that perhaps there are some optometrists who talk about "The Core Philosophy" much as Danny gave impressive lip service to the Pledge of Allegiance.

Fully realizing that my comments here may add to the confusion more than moving us toward clarification, I must attempt to look at the meaning at the relevancies of "the Core Philosophy" as it pertains to what we hold as a central theme. Recognizing all the risks that lie in this attempt, it seems most appropriate we start with an exploration of the several flat, oft repeated phrases that outline "The Core Philosophy." Skeffington called these phrases "notions" but Mr. Webster gives us the word "dogma" that he defines as "1a. something held as an established opinion, 1b. a code of such tenets, 1c. a point of view, or tenet, put forth as authoritative without adequate grounds." Thus, Webster's choice leads to my use of the word dogma.

Dogma #1: "Vision is the dominant process in human behavior."

This short statement, credited to Arnold Gesell, M.D., (one of the most prominent of all developmentalists) slips off the tongue of many optometrist as if it were a hard and fully established fact. The only fact that really exists here is that his was an opinion, easily believed and expressed by us because it is so supportive to the concepts held by we behavioral optometrists. There is ample, fully validated scientific data to support this opinion but we must constantly remind ourselves that no matter how valid the scientific evidence, the dominance is neither innate nor a certainty for every individual. One can easily defend this notion of dominancy if the statement is rephrased: "vision will become the most dominant process in human behavior when all developmental processes expand and organize according to their innate design." This is not a quibbling statement as a substitute for the original statement by Gesell. It is just a more realistic expression of the genetic design, and the events that allow vision to become the most significant and effective of all the information processing systems when adequate development does occur in the full course of reaching for the ultimate potential present in the human. This restatement allows for the factual and valid examples of individuals in whom the visual process does not become the dominant influence in their behavior, with performance levels below the potentials, which would have been reached IF vision had become the dominant process.

This revision of Dogma #1 is essential to the realistic comprehensions, which guide the behavioral optometrist. It must be clinically recognized that if vision has not achieved its innately expected performance levels, the behavioral optometrist cannot expect to guide such a patient to the ultimate visual skills by employing selected, specific attacks on the visual system in degrees of isolation. If one, or more, of the other information processing systems has achieved a level of dominance (or preference) the behavioral optometrist must be totally aware of, and employ, the regimens that will permit the patient to move through his, or her, established preferences so the individual may then move toward the dominance of the visual system that is so essential to the social and economic survival in the present culture, now so symbolically loaded.

This, if "The Core Philosophy" is to truly include Dogma #1, the behavioral optometrist must fully recognize the contributions each of the relevant systems do provide to vision development. This is not to imply that the behavioral optometrist becomes fully informed in the anatomy, neurology, and physiology of each of the contributing systems, but there must be the general understanding of what each can, and will, contribute to the emergent we call vision. Of equal importance is the understanding of how these contributions can be clinically integrated into visual performance for the extension and elaborations of the visual system. There must be much more than lip service given to the roles of the other systems. There must be a clear understanding of their contributions and their limitations, and how other systems must fit into the visual process if it is to reach the role in behavior, which is attributed to it. For example: if the tactual system (commonly the manual touch actions) is to make its contributions to vision, it must bring much more than mere contact. It must contribute qualities of object and/or symbol size, shape, texture, weight, solidity and temperature which can then be translated by the visual system into visual interpretations that will eventually replace, or mediate, touch. Or, if the auditory system is to be a contributor, the signals from audition must contain those special characteristics, which will contribute to spatial orientations, which are common to vision. The mere rhythm of a metronome is not enough of a signal for audition to make its contribution. Noise must come from a spatial position that can be identified visually, or noise is nothing more than noise and will have no visual qualities.

Perhaps all of this comes down to the final comprehension of what the behavioral optometrist means when the word dominant (or dominance) is used. This word must not negate all other information systems in every interpretive action. What it should mean is that the visual system can, and should, become the carrier, the integrator and synthesizer, for all of the information all the other systems can contribute to the ultimate comprehension of all those bits of information out of the lighted world which the individual can then catalyze into intellectual growth and behavior. As a result of this process just described, that is unique to vision, the intellectual processes can operate with speed and efficiency, which will bring an individual to an ultimate level of human behavior.

Dogma #2: "Since vision is learned and developed, vision is trainable."

This statement can best be attributed to Prof. Sam Renshaw, experimental psychologist, of Ohio State University until the late 1960s. This is another of the statements that have become glibly expressed clichés among optometrist. No matter how much clinical evidence there is to support this statement, it is still the point of greatest controversy – both outside and (unfortunately) inside of optometry. It seems the major point of contention arises because there is still so much confusion over what we optometrists mean when we say the word vision. It is very obvious to many of us that those who condemn this statement are still thinking of sight and vision as interchangeable terms describing the visual act. A philosophy that still holds the classical medical-camera model (what I call the *medicam* model) as sufficient to explain the reception and interpretations of what is seen, can never accept that vision is learned, or that it can be more adequately developed.

The idea that clarity of sight is the only criterion required to appraise visual abilities will forever limit any understanding of visual performance. Only when one realizes that what we call acuity is much more dependent upon experience than it is on some sort of retinal imagery will there be any freedom to understand the learning process, which is so intimately related to visual interpretations. As we optometrists observe infant visual behavior we are consistently struck with the infant's visual attention to minute details of those objects with which there is familiarity. The non-optometric contention that "visual acuities" are not "neurologically" possible until after several years of life continue to confuse the issue primarily because the ancient textbooks simply have not been updated as a direct result of wide and indisputable studies of the infant's visual performance.

The behavioral optometrist would profit from some revision of this persistent cliché. Much of the confusion and contention could be eliminated if we would state, "The skills of visual inspection, discrimination and interpretation are learned through actual experience and practice. Thus, these visual skills are trainable as are all other learned skills." Even the most insistent contradictor would have difficulty denying this statement.

Dogma #3 "Vision and intelligence are one and the same."

This statement slipped off the tongue of Professor Ward Halstead, of Chicago University until the late 1970s, as he lectured to optometrists at the Heart of America Congress in Kansas City, Missouri, late in the 1950s. The interesting fact here is that this very astute bio-neuro-psychologist understood vision as we in behavioral optometry understood it. Professor Halstead's close friendship with A.M. Skeffington, and other optometrists, brought his deep understanding of mental functions to the assistance of those of us striving to understand vision. It was probably the use of the retinoscope in the observations of "comprehension" that most attracted Halstead's interest. After his personal experiences with optometric retinoscopic observations on himself, and on his Chicago University graduate students, Halstead commented as he did.

Unfortunately, all those who equate sight and vision are immediately shocked with such a dogmatic statement. Thus, their shock is understandable, and this is another phrase that some revision would improve. Perhaps, if was stated it, "Since visual discriminations and interpretations are so critical to comprehension, visual skills can make significant contributions to intellectual conclusions. If so, then visual skills can be significant contributors to intelligence, and intellectual behavior." Perhaps, also, such revision will clarify this particular dogma as an important part of "The Core Philosophy."

Dogma #4: "Positive changes in visual behavior will only occur when there is the full implementation, and organization, of movement abilities."

Although A.M. Skeffington, with his amazing foresight, included movement as a critical factor in visual organization (his "antigravity" circle), the full appreciation of movement came from the contributions of Darell Boyd Harmon, Ph.D., -- that most amazing neuro-bio-psycho-physiological educationist who came into the optometric picture in the early 50s. Early in the development of "The Core Philosophy" movement was credited mostly with its influence upon bilaterality and the extended influence upon development and functions of binocularity. This early emphasis upon movement as a part of optometric vision training regimens was twofold: to get the optometric patient out of the restricting stereo instruments used while seated, and into what we then called "free space", and to get an interweaving of the two sides of the body as a more adequate supporting structure for development of bi-ocularity as it was described by Gesell and his staff. The great contribution from Harmon was the realization that movement was the major contributor to the organization of the individual's mastery of visual space for egocentric orientations from which all visual decisions could then be made.

There is more and more literature appearing in which human movement, and its purpose, is discussed. Interestingly, most of this literature continues to consider movement as the primary sensorimotor complex that is sufficient unto itself in the organization of human behavior. As an optometrist, fully indoctrinated on the significance of vision and its roles in both feedback and feed forward of spatial information, it is difficult to read this splendid literature and to accept the author's omission of vision as the ultimate monitor and modifier of all movement – no matter what its origin or purpose.

Once again, any statement on the importance of movement as the genesis of experience, which is to become the genesis of intelligence, must include the visual system as its director, monitor and modifier. Thus, the statement given here as Dogma #4 should be rephrased: "Positive changes in visual behavior will only occur when there is the full exploration of movement abilities that are consistently directed, monitored and mediated by visual discriminations and the decisions which follow such visual discriminations." If "The Core Philosophy" is to be a valid and viable outline for behavioral optometry then there must be the realization that movement for movement's sake will not bring the changes in visual organization we seek for the patient. ONLY that movement that has vision as its guide and appraiser will be of developmental value to the patient, and only that movement which demands changes in the visual interpretations of one's position in lighted space will bring the desired changes in the visual organization of the patient. It is here that lenses and prisms will have the significant impact as these insist upon changes in the visual interpretations of posture and position. A rebounder (ed. trampoline) for rebounding is nothing more than gymnastic exercise, and cannot be construed to be an optometric procedure. If a rebounder is to be used, there most be some sort of visual decisions about one's spatial position and the postural changes this induced. Only if there are these visual contemplations can the rebounder become an optometric instrument with legality in "The Core Philosophy."

Dogma #5: "Lenses and prisms must be consistently used by the patient if the desired changes in visual behavior are to be achieved."

A few years ago this statement was issued as a primary rule of all visual training procedures. It created considerable discussion because many optometrists contended that there are times when lenses had either no influence upon the ocularmotor system, or had no purpose – as in "closed eye" procedures, or in visualization routines. Such a contention is understandable if one's model is limited to what lenses, and/or prisms, do to the optics of the eyes.

The lifelong work of Harmon, and many of his protégés clearly and indisputably shows that the impact of lenses and prisms is first, and most emphatically, upon posture – and that the resulting changes in postural signals then influence the response to the lenses and prism. All of this returns us to Skeffington's second circle which he called <u>centering</u>, and which some optometrists unfortunately limited to <u>convergence</u>, and vergences in general. Again, Skeffington in his amazing foresight was presenting the word centering as the process of spatial orientations. Harmon then came along to impress upon all of us that spatial orientations were the direct product of posture. I would like to submit to you the possibility that if one visualizes orientational space outward this could have the same perceptual result as a plus lens, or base in prisms. If one visualizes orientational space inward this could have the same perceptual result as a minus lens, or base out prisms. If retinoscopy was possible through closed lids, I would wager that there could be observed those refractive changes which come from lenses and prisms before open eyes, and, I will wager these visualizations will bring postural changes.

Now, as we behavioral optometrist head into another decade of searching for a fuller understanding of the total visual process, we must understand that "The Core Philosophy" holds lenses and prisms as optometry's unique tool to change spatial judgments and decisions, and out of these will come the actions of the end organs that we measure with all our special probes and observations. In some manner, if we are to expand and extend the concepts set out for us by Skeffington and his associates over the past 60 years, we must come to the understanding of what the old law holds – that functions will influence structure more than structure will influence function. Only thus, can we begin to understand what Skeffington was repeatedly stating when he insisted that visual problems would eventually bring ocular problems. As we finally achieve this understanding we will then begin to appreciate why lenses and prisms must be a consistent part of all optometric prescriptions – for visual development, training, prevention, enhancement, and lastly, compensation.

Dogma #6: "The complete Skeffington Analytical Sequence is the only true appraisal of visual abilities."

The accuracy of this statement depends upon what information the appraiser wants. If the refractive status – traditionally called the "refractive error" – is all the clinician wants to determine, then the Skeffington Analytical Sequence (SAS) takes "too much time" and, yes, "there are easier ways to do it." If, in high contrast, the optometric clinician wants to know how effectively and successfully a patient performs in meeting the demands the culture puts on the individual, then the SAS is the only sequence of interrelated probes and observations that will provide the essential information. The "refractive error" search will determine the lens powers for 20/20 clarity for most general distance visual tasks – and little else. The SAS will provide the same detail, but only as one small detail in the total appraisal of how well the selected lenses will allow the patient to effectively and successfully master his, or her, environment and all of the visual challenges it presents.

These past few years have brought numerous remarks about the need for revisions and replacements for the SAS. Those who most frequently insist upon these changes also insist only part of the sequence is needed to determine the most suitable lens prescription. This may be true if the lens prescription is the only purpose of the evaluation. If the patient's total visual performance, and its influence upon total behavior, is the purpose of the optometric evaluation, then every probe in the sequence should be carefully included because every one of the 21 probes has a clinical reason, and will provide information that should not be ignored. Perhaps we must consider the possibility that the foreshortening of the evaluation routine is not because of shortcomings of the SAS but is a sign of a lack of full understanding of the SAS and the values it contains. This apparent lack of understanding more and more frequently shows up in the brevity of the case records being exhibited by some optometrist. In numerous instances, probes are omitted that would serve as baseline information for the analysis of performance on the other probes. Or, some probes are included as if they need no comparison, or equation, with related probes. One of the greatest values of the SAS is the basic design wherein every probe in the series is intimately related to another probe. It is the full appreciation of these relationships that makes the sequence such a true appraisal of human visual abilities. The optometrist who insists the entire SAS is not needed is missing the opportunity to fully appreciate the visual organization the patient brings into the examining room – and the applications the patient makes of this visual organization out in his, or her, lighted world.

This statement might be then expanded to read: "The Skeffington Analytical Sequence is the only true appraisal of visual abilities <u>as these influence a patient in his, or her occupational and avocational environment</u>." As of this moment, no one has presented a replacement for the SAS that will serve the purposes it serves. If, and when, someone does offer an adequate substitute even the most persistent of the SAS supporters will welcome it as a contribution to daily clinical demands. Until then, "The Core Philosophy" will continue to include the complete Skeffington Analytical Sequence as its baseline appraisal of human visual performance and the behavior it produces.

It does not take much analysis to determine that the common thread running through these six points of delineation is the totality of the organism, and the primary role that vision plays in all productive human behavior. The grasp an optometrist has on this central theme will not be evidenced simply by agreement with the dogmas just described. It certainly is not a question of whether or not the optometrist agrees that vision is the dominant process in human behavior; or that vision is developed and learned and thus is trainable; or that vision and intelligence are one and the same; or that movement abilities determine visual abilities; or that lenses and prisms are the essential implement for changes in human behavior as these influence posture; or that the complete SAS is the only way to appraise visual abilities. These dogmas are nothing more than descriptions of the foundational tenets of behavioral optometry. The final depth of the grasp one achieves on this philosophy will be evidenced by what one judges as the final criterion of visual abilities and visual performance. As has already been stated, all of the neuro-physiological components must be recognized and understood for the implementation of the covert processes these dogmas suggest. It will be the recognition and understanding of when, how, and where overt human behavior is the output of these processes that will determine how extensively the optometrist sees the role that vision plays in the patient's mastery of the lighted environment which surrounds him, or her. As Skeffington so often implied it: the light from the environment creates the input; the processing and organization of all the covert processes which act upon this input will be the put-put, and the observable behavior of the individual as a result of both the input and put-put will be the output we behavioral optometrists must learn to more fully appreciate. When the appreciation is finally achieved, there will come the understanding of all the sub-factors, which will permit the release of the "medicam model" that has trapped the traditionalists for so many decades.

What then IS "The Core Philosophy" so frequently acclaimed by behavioral optometrists? Perhaps, if we are to follow the advice of the ancient Chinese philosopher in finding a "proper name" – or to hear Secretary Shultz's suggestion that we "rectify names" – we will find a better label for the concepts we hold. If we find a better label might we also find better understandings? Would it not be more fully descriptive, and more expressive if we just simply called the theme we hold, "The behavioral philosophy for optometry"? It seems to me this would more accurately stakes out and identifies all of the aspects of the central theme I have just discussed. I am personally already finding this is much more comfortable for me, and I submit to this idea to you for your consideration.

Nearpoint Lens Prescriptions: Clinical Methods for Comparing and Evaluating Selected Dynamic Retinoscopy Techniques

Harold M. Haynes, O.D.
Forest Grove, OR

Introduction

Selected dynamic retinoscopy procedures were discussed at the 17th annual meeting of the COVD in Philadelphia in November, 1987. Four optometrists were invited to review their contributions and hold a workshop to demonstrate their methods and procedures. The invited participants in order of presentation and topics were: Doctors G.N. Getman, Book Retinoscopy; H.M. Haynes, Combined MEMLN Retinoscopy; R.J. Apell, Bell Retinoscopy; and R. Kraskin, Stresspoint Retinoscopy.

During the question and answer period, a great deal of interest was expressed by the audience as to how these retinoscopy procedures could be used to write a Nearpoint lens prescription for infants, children and adults. Dr. Nathan Flax asked Haynes to compare the similarities and differences in a lens prescription which would result from using the several methods of retinoscopy presented. To elaborate on Flax's question, assume four different optometrists independently examined the same patient, each using one of the four different retinoscopy techniques. Assume further, that each examiner was skilled in the technique and agreed to write a spherical lens prescription based solely on the dynamic retinoscopy observations as recommended by the authorities above. Diagnostically, would each examiner find a lens prescription indicated? How would the lens prescriptions, if any, compare?

This paper is a serious attempt to answer theoretically Professor Flax's question based on our present knowledge. Ideally, the answers to the several questions raised above should be provided by controlled clinical trials. In the absence of an appropriate clinical study, I will use existing information to examine theoretically the several clinical problems which are involved with predicting the outcome if such an empirical study was undertaken. As will be seen, this theoretical analysis would be necessary even if a controlled experiment were contemplated or actually performed.

Separation of Problems

Four problem areas are analyzed theoretically for comparative purposes. These four separable and interrelated problem areas are:
1. Similarities and differences in administering the specific retinoscopy techniques.
2. Diagnostic uses and limits with each of the techniques.
3. Conversion of quantitative measurements within and among the techniques. Simple models developed to allow MEM observations to be converted to expected Book, Bell or Stresspoint measurements and vice versa as a result of different testing distances.
4. Similarities and differences in lens prescriptions resulting from the several procedures.

Historically, Getman [1,2], in his pioneering work at the Gesell Institute, introduced Book retinoscopy, also called cognitive retinoscopy, as a means of observing dynamic refractive changes of the eye when infants and children were shown a wide range of targets with books and pictures under many different instructional sets, states and observational conditions. Initially, the procedure was not designed to quantitatively determine a nearpoint lens prescription. The Monocular Estimate Method (MEM) was introduced initially by Haynes [3], at Pacific University, primarily as a diagnostic tool to control unwanted optical variables associated with Book retinoscopy and to determine if a nearpoint prescription was indicated. By observing proper controls and target selection, effects of variables associated with angular size, distance, target complexity, symbolic significance, tasks and instructions can be isolated and evaluated for clinical purposes. Apell [4,5] and his co-worker Streff, [6] working at the Gesell Institute, and Kraskin, [7,8] in his own office; have developed slightly differing hetero-dynamic procedures from different theoretical assumptions which are quite useful for both diagnostic and quantitative determination of a new lens prescription. Apell refers to his technique as Bell retinoscopy and Kraskin describes his as Stresspoint. More recently, Haynes has combined the MEM with Sheard's Low Neutral retinoscopy [9,10] [LN] procedure. The Combined MEM-LN[11] procedure was designed to improve physiological understanding of accommodative performance by isolating specific motor and refractive variables which are necessary for increased understanding and better design of nearpoint lens prescriptions. When used without lenses, the original MEM observations alone are not considered theoretically adequate for quantitative determination of a nearpoint lens.

Overview of Techniques

The similarities and differences in testing procedures among the several dynamic retinoscopy procedures are summarized briefly below. This summary includes only the degree of detail which is required for the theoretical analysis which follows. For detailed descriptions, see the writings of the individual authorities.

Each of the procedures may be performed without any lenses, through the patient's habitual prescription, through the distance subjective refraction or any other lens control the examiner desires. Unless stated otherwise, for simplification of the theoretical analysis the best measurable distance refraction, including aniso and cylinder, measured from the accommodative endpoint [*punctum remotum* of accommodation] is assumed as a control. Thus, "optically induced emmetropia" may be assumed for analysis purposes. Where necessary, examples of hyperopes and myopes wearing no lenses will be discussed.

Book

Eye to task distance: Various distances have been reported including approximately 40 cm for adults, at an individual's Harmon distance and at a child's selected reading distance when holding the book. The retinoscope is located as close to top of book as possible to attempt to control "off axis" or oblique retinoscopy and to have approximately the same eye to retinoscope aperture distance as eye to task distance.

Target: Story book with pictures suitable for age, paragraph reading, etc.

Retinoscopy observation: The examiner records changes in color, brightness and estimates average magnitude and differences in motion as the instructed task is performed [Motion = with, against, neutral, spherical, irregular and/or astigmatic]. When motion is to be quantitatively measured, a lens equal to the examiner's estimate is brought before one eye for as short a time as possible until neutral is observed. Getman, when observing changes in color, brightness and the light pattern in the entire reflex used a stationary retinoscope rather than the sweeping scan used to observe motion.

MEM
Eye to task and retinoscope to eye distances are controlled by fastening the target to retinoscope. The ideal installation of the target plane would be at the retinoscope aperture plane distance.

Target: Test cards, instructions and norms are standardized for 40 cm [16 inches]. Test figures on each test card have a maximum subtended angle of 5 degrees or less from a line perpendicular from the center of the retinoscope aperture. Observations at other distances may be readily computed and compared with 40cm responses so long as the subtended angles do not exceed 5°.

Retinoscopy observation: Starting with the retinoscope light on the bridge of the nose, both eyes are alternately scanned by the retinoscope. Motion is estimated whenever possible to eliminate the vergence from the neutralizing lens from becoming part of the accommodative stimulus and thus changing the accommodative response. Estimated motion is checked by monocular introduction of a neutralizing lens for the shortest time possible. Emphasis is on estimation of motion rather than color and/or brightness changes because no valid quantitative standards for scaling have been published to date.

Bell
Eye to task distance: In most cases, eye to task distance is varied and retinoscope to eye distance is held at a constant 50 cm [20 inches].

Target: Dangled bell or smooth steel ball mounted on a rod. Either fixation target is hand held by retinoscopist. The patient is instructed to constantly fixate the bell which is initially held at the same distance as the retinoscope.

Retinoscopy observation: The retinoscopist alternately sweeps each eye. When "with" motion is seen, the bell is moved towards the patient on the midline until the initially observed "with" motion is reduced to a "neutral" motion. The eye to fixation target [bell] distance is measured. If the eye to target distance is significantly less than 38 to 40 cm [15 to 16 inches] then plus spheres are added binocularity in 0.25D or 0.50D steps until the eye to fixation target approximates 15" to 16" on repeated measurements. The magnitude of the lenses before each eye becomes the suggested value for the nearpoint spherical lens prescription.

Stresspoint

The procedure is the same as Bell retinoscopy except that Kraskin recommends a stationary retinoscope observation of each eye. This technique uses criteria different than first-observable-neutral as the endpoint for measuring the eye to fixation target distance. A sudden dimming followed by an immediate maximum brightening of the reflex is described as the "stress point" hence the name. [Editor's note: This is exactly the opposite of the observations as published in *Lens Power in Action* by Robert A. Kraskin. We do not know if Haynes simply misstated it here or if there was a misunderstanding at a different level.] The brief dimming before maximum brightening of the brightness may not be observable. In personal communications with Dr. Kraskin, he states that based on his clinical observations that the two procedures usually yield about the same lens power. When the two procedures differ, the stresspoint criterion averages about a 0.25D more plus than Bell. Kraskin's observations seem theoretically consistent. With a stationary retinoscope, an observed difference in maximum brightness and a "full pupil" of light would be expected optically to occur just before or after neutral is observed with a moving retinoscope.

Combined MEM-LN

The MEM portion of the procedure is performed as described above when a circular array of 20/100 letters is read orally slowly by the patient Depending on the magnitude of the initial "with" motion during the MEM observation, plus spheres are added binocularly in 0.25D or 0.50D steps until first neutral and first against motion is observed. With each successive addition of plus spheres the motion is estimated and recorded. The results are treated mathematically and/or graphed and compared to published patterns of response to understand the mode of accommodative response to change in lenses and to obtain a nearpoint prescription. The degree of relative accommodative tracking is observed. See Figure 1 for an example of plotting the several measurements.

PLOTTING TECHNIQUE FOR COMBINED MEM-LN RETINOSCOPY

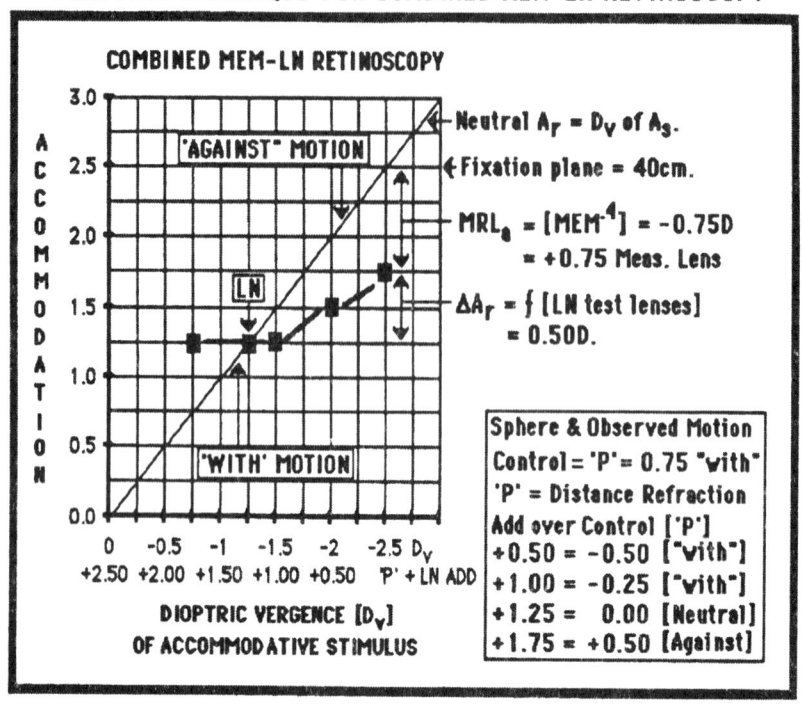

Figure 1. MEM-LN isodynamic retinoscopy. Vertical axis is a plot of the accommodative response as measured by dynamic retinoscopy where the distance refraction ['P'] is set equal to zero [0.00D]. Horizontal axis plot contains the reciprocal of the distance in meters, the dioptric vergence [D_v] of the wavefront of the accommodative stimulus; and the Low Neutral [LN] plus sphere add values over 'P'. "With" motion is plotted below the diagonal line and "Against" motion is plotted above the diagonal. A "Neutral" motion is plotted on the line indicating that accommodation plus the dioptric value of the spherical test lenses are focused in the aperture plane of the retinoscope. In this example, accommodation is postured -0.75D behind the fixation plane at 40cm through the distance refraction and -1.25D beyond with a +1.25D sphere [LN]. The change in the accommodative response [ĊAr] is a 0.50D as a function of 1.25D reduction in the accommodative stimulus.

Book, when optical variables are controlled, MEM, and the Combined MEM-LN procedures are classified as essentially isodynamic techniques indicating that the retinoscope aperture and the target plane are approximately coincident. Bell and Stresspoint are hetero-dynamic procedures indicating that the retinoscope aperture is remote from the fixation target. Quantification of retinoscopic observations with isodynamic procedures involved either estimating the motion, and/or using the monocular introduction of spheres to check the estimate; or binocular introduction of spheres before both eyes until no motion in seen such as in low and high neutral techniques. Whenever spheres are introduced, they change the stimulus to accommodation and usually change the accommodative response. Hetero-dynamic procedures are quantified quite accurately by determining the dioptric difference between the plane of the fixation target and the eye and the retinoscope aperture to eye distance. This dioptric difference becomes a direct measure of the motor response lag of accommodation [MRL_a] at that distance [specific definition later].

Diagnostic Considerations

Assuming the distal endpoint refraction is used as a control or that the patient is emmetropic, let us consider how and to what extent the following information may be extracted from the several retinoscopy procedures described above. Consider the following question sets:

1. Is a nearpoint lens prescription indicated? Is it the same or different than the control lens? Distance refraction?
2. If a new lens is indicated and prescribed, how will image definition be changed?
3. If a new lens is indicated and prescribed, what is the estimated magnitude in the change of the accommodative response? Probable interactive effect on convergence?
4. For any given retinoscopy technique, how do we operationally define such physiological and optical constructs as accommodative response, accommodative posture relative to the fixation plane, accommodative lag, etc?
5. Under these clinical test conditions, what are the significant stimulus and response variables which control the accommodative response? What generalizations can be safely made relative to accommodative performance during various normal visual tasks?

Based on current knowledge, the above retinoscopy techniques may be expected to show general agreement by identifying those cases requiring a nearpoint lens prescription based on observable accommodative disturbances. This same generalization is probably true for low hyperopes measured with no lenses but is not applicable for myopes wearing no lenses. On myopes, near findings should be taken with both the habitual state and the farpoint refraction as a control. Conversely, depending on the prescription criterion used, these retinoscopy procedures may, on selected cases, yield a wide range of prescriptions from a +0.25D to +2.00D add at 16". To illustrate these opinions, assume the following findings for two hypothetical patients A and B who are examined with the targets and techniques described above. Assume valid and reliable measurements in the findings below.

Patient A: Book = 0.25D to 0.50D "with" MEM = stable 0.50D "with." Bell = 17" [43cm]. Stresspoint = 16" [40cm]. Low Neutral [LN] = +1.00D add; first "against" = +1.75D @ 16".

Patient B: Book = dull, variable "with," ranging from 0.75D to 1.50D. MEM = 1.00 to 1.50D "with". Bell = 10.5" [~27cm]. Stresspoint = 10" [25cm]. Low Neutral [LN] = +1.75D add; first "against" = +2.00D @ 16".

Based on the published standards, Patient A would require no near add, or lenses, based on the findings given. Bell and Stresspoint are considered within the desired range for "normal" performance. The "with" motion on Book and MEM at 40cm is likewise considered "normal" because it is less than the .075D "with" decision point. By normative standards, the accommodative lag, the motor response lag of accommodation, the accommodative posture measured from the fixation plane and the accommodative response are all rated as normal to superior given the gross targets used for testing. [The several descriptive terms just used are operationally defined in the next section under "Conversion Calculations."] Image formation is considered adequate for most every day discriminatory tasks. Fine discriminatory tasks at 40cm would require about a 0.25D increase in response for 40cm over the gross target response.

Conversely, Patient B indicates a nearpoint prescription if the patient's lifestyle includes sustained nearpoint activities with and/or without asthenopic symptoms. The observed "with" motion in both Book and

MEM average will above acceptable levels for gross targets. Bell and Stresspoint eye to target distances are well inside the 15" to 16" range of normalcy. Image definition is degraded when looking at gross targets and should be increasingly so with a further decrease in fixation distance. Fine discriminatory tasks at 40cm would require an increase of about 1.00D of accommodation. Hypo-posturing accommodation is evident as is the abnormal motor response lag of accommodation.

Question sets 3 and 5 above can be only partially answered with the data given. Quantitative determination of the change in accommodation from a lens prescription requires the data from the Combined MEM-LN procedure to answer Q3. Question 5, dealing with identification of significant elements of the accommodative stimulus can only be answered by systematically testing the MEM responses with carefully designed targets, standardized instructions and specific discriminatory tasks to explore these variables. This last statement is equally true for the other retinoscopy techniques. To my knowledge, neither Apell, Getman nor Kraskin has developed a target series to isolate the controlling stimulus elements. I plan to address this aspect of my own work in a future paper.

Conversion Calculations

A reasonable level of patient management can be achieved from treating cases diagnostically as exemplified above by following an authority's recommendation for a specific test or procedure. However, detailed comparative analysis of accommodative performance involving evaluation of the results from different lens prescriptions criteria requires additional quantitative and theoretical tools. Underlying assumptions and prescription criteria need to be detailed specifically for theoretical analysis. To begin an expanded theoretical analysis, simple models are presented below to transpose a specific finding measured at one distance to a second distance or to convert MEM measurements into Bell or Stresspoint or vice versa. Such conversions are necessary for comparative review of the literature or for the study of an individual case where multiple retinoscopy procedures are used.

Assumptions: The simple mathematical and graphical conversion models which follow are based on the following three assumptions. (1) It is assumed that when optical, target, task and instructional variables are controlled; the response of accommodation as a function of changing fixation distance is linear over a range from about 20cm to 1 meter provided the amplitude of accommodation is equal to or greater than 6 diopters. (2) It is assumed that the accommodative response will be approximately equal in magnitude with the bell, the steel ball, the circular 20/100 letter target and the 20/350 number target when distance, task and instructions are similar. (3) It is assumed that the "neutral" motion endpoint in Bell retinoscopy is equivalent to Kraskin's endpoint in Stresspoint retinoscopy.

Support for the three assumptions cited above includes: Previous reported studies show that MEM, LN, and HM dynamic procedures are linear at near distances when task and target conditions are controlled. See Figure 2. Further, by computing the mean values for the accommodative lag at 40cm from Apell's and Kraskin's recommended prescription distances and comparing these figures with average MEM value for 20/350 digit reading and 20/100 letter reading it seems safe to conclude that the bell, steel ball and the two acuity targets all yield similar mean dioptric values. This conclusion is further supported because these mean values are in accord with Sheard's and Tait's values, among many others, for 40cm. It would be very helpful if correlations were available to further define the similarities. If Book retinoscopy is performed with the same controls, targets and instructions and at the same distance[s] as the MEM procedure the results will be the same. When different results were obtained, I have found without exception that the differences have arisen from uncontrolled optical or physical variables. Until evidence to the contrary is presented, and based on personal communications with Kraskin, Bell and Stresspoint techniques will be considered equivalent for theoretical computational purposes.

MULTIPLE DISTANCE DYNAMIC RETINOSCOPY

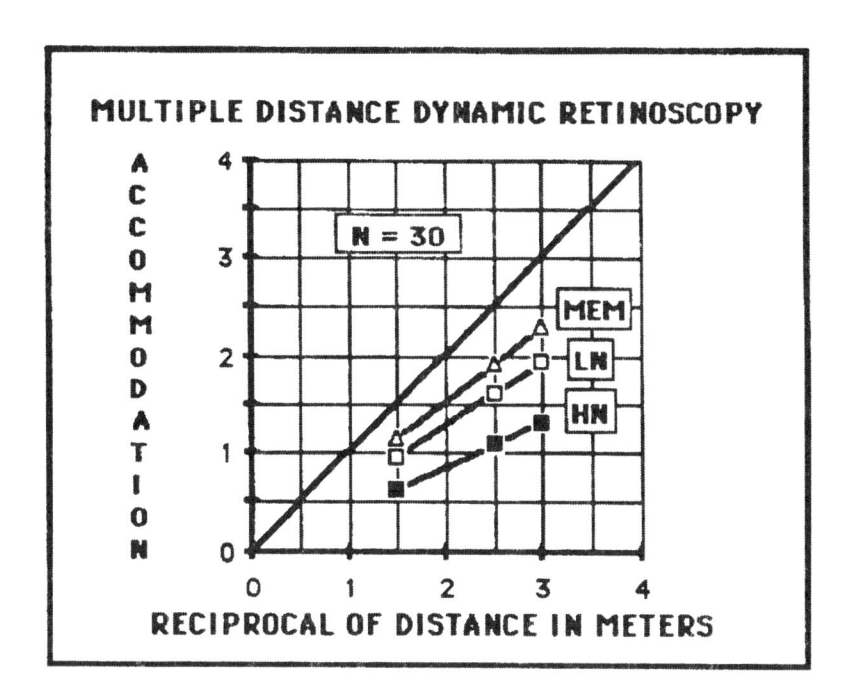

(Graph: ACCOMMODATION vs RECIPROCAL OF DISTANCE IN METERS, N = 30, showing three curves labeled MEM, LN, and HN)

Figure 2 Mean accommodative response as a function of changing fixation distance with MEM, LN and HN testing conditions. The response of accommodation to the test lenses is indicated by the displacement of the three linear curves from 33cm to 67cm. The slopes of the three curves for the three procedures are significantly different.

For purposes of this paper and the computations which follow, the following terms and symbols are defined as they apply to dynamic retinoscopy. Calculations for Patient's A & B follow these definitions.

Let the symbol **'P'** = any valid distal endpoint [*punctum remotum*] for distance refraction. 'P' is used as the metric zero point for measurement of the distal accommodative endpoint.

Accommodative response [A_r] = accommodation measured in diopters by retinoscopy or valid optometer from 'P'. Objective change in eye dioptrics is measured from the *punctum remotum* of accommodation.

Accommodative posture [Ap] = locus of accommodation in diopters measured in response units proximally or distally from the fixation plane rather than from the distal endpoint ['P'].

Accommodative lag [A$_L$] = the difference obtained when 'P' is subtracted from any gross near dynamic retinoscopy test measured in diopters with a given fixation distance. Examples: A$_L$ = [MEM – P] or [LN – P] etc. These differences are measurement units. In response units (eye dioptrics) the signs are reversed. A$_L$ = [P – MEM] or [P – LN] or any other dynamic retinoscopy.

Motor response lag of accommodation [MRL$_a$] = dioptrics difference between the dioptrics vergence [D$_v$] of the wavefront of the combined accommodative stimulus from lenses and fixation distance and the accommodative response. MRL$_a$ = [D$_v$ + A$_r$]. Where D$_v$ = 1/d + lens vergence. And, where 1/d = the reciprocal of the distance in meters. International sign conventions are used to specify wavefront [D$_v$].

From the assumptions and definitions above, it can be shown that when, and only when, any of the dynamic retinoscopy procedures are taken through the distance refraction 'P'; the accommodative posture, the accommodative lag and the motor response lag of accommodation will have the same dioptrics value [Ap = AL = MRLa] at the same distance. When any other spherical values are used for testing, these values may be different depending on the test conditions. Hence, the theoretical need for the three descriptive terms often included under the single tern "accommodative lag".

Figure 2 displays mean dynamic retinoscopy data at near for MEM, Low Neutral [LN] and high Neutral [HN] procedures. The linear results and the differences in the three curves are the result of the preset conditions and more specifically the plus spheres used to measure LN and HN retinoscopy. The test lenses change the vergence of the accommodative stimulus with a resultant change in accommodative response. Bell and Stresspoint, when measured through the distance retinoscopy finding are expected to fall on the MEM curve.

To predict the expected [estimated] value for any nearpoint isodynamic retinoscopy at another distance when the first test was taken through the distance refraction, 'P', requires computing a lag/distance ratio. The numerator is the dioptrics value of any isodynamic retinoscopy finding in add form. The denominator of the ratio is the reciprocal of the eye to task distance measured in meters. For example suppose 0.25D "with" motion is observed with MEM at 40cm. Lag/distance ratio is obtained by dividing the reciprocal of 40cm in meters into 0.25D. Result: [0.25 ÷ 2.5] = 0.1. To predict the estimated value of an isodynamic retinoscopy for a different near distance, multiply the lag/distance ratio times the reciprocal of the new fixation distance in meters. This, when lag/distance ratio = .1, the expected values [$_e$MRL$_a$] for 50cm = 0.20D, for 33cm = 0.30D, for 25cm = 0.40D and for 20cm = 0.50D. And, if the MEM at 40cm – 1.25 "with", then, lag/distance ratio is [1.25 ÷ 2.5] = 0.5. The expected values [$_e$MRL$_a$] for 50cm – 1.00D, for 33cm = 1.50D, for 25cm = 2.00D and for 20cm = 2.50D. LN and HN estimates are calculated in the same manner.

To compare Bell/Stresspoint hetero-dynamic to isodynamic procedures [MEM,LN,HN] requires three steps. [i] The MRL$_a$ is obtained by obtaining the difference in diopters between the reciprocal of the retinoscope to eye distance and the target to eye distance. Example: Neutral motion is observed when the bell target is at 10 inches [25cm] and the retinoscope aperture is at 20 inches [50cm]. The MRL$_a$ is a - 2.00D, [1/.5 – 1/.25 = -2.00D] at 25cm. [ii] The lag/distance ratio is calculated as described in the paragraph above. This, in the example with the -2.00D MRL$_a$, the lag/distance ratio is 0.5, [2.00 ÷ 1/.25 = 0.5]. The lag/distance ratio for the MEM and the Bell/Stresspoint responses are then compared. Or, if desired, if the MEM is in diopters at 40cm, the $_e$MRL$_a$ for 40cm can be calculated and compared to the empirical measurement. The $_e$MRL$_a$ at 40cm in our example is -1.25D, [.5 x 1/.4 = 1.25].

Patient A's findings are quantified as follows. Since our hypothetical cases were taken through the distance refraction ['P'] the A$_p$, A$_L$, and MRL$_a$ values at 40cm in response terms all indicate that accommodation is behind the fixation plane. The average dioptrics values for the observations are: Book = -0.37D. MEM = -0.50D. Stresspoint = -0.50D. Bell = -0.33D. In the first three tests fixation was at 40cm. In Bell, the fixation distance was 43 cm [17"]. The average dioptrics values for the accommodative response [A$_r$ = 1/d + A$_L$] are: Book [2.5+ (-0.37)] = 2.12D. MEM [2.5 + (-0.50)] = 2.00D. Stresspoint [2.5 + (+0.50)] = 2.00D. Bell [2.33 + (-0.33)] = 2.00D.

Bell and Stresspoint values above are obtained by converting eye to retinoscopy and eye to task distances [fixation distance] to diopters [1/d in meters]. The dioptrics interval between the bell and the plane of the retinoscope aperture is the quantitative measure of the magnitude that the accommodative response lags or leads the fixation target. This interval is a direct measure of the MRL_a.

For Patient B, the average dioptrics values for the A_p, A_L, and MRL_a values are: Book = -1.12D. MEM = -1.25D. Stresspoint = -2.00D. Bell = -1.70D. The average dioptrics values for the accommodative response $[A_r = 1/d + A_L]$ are: Book [2.5 = (-1.12)] = 1.37D. MEM [2.5 + (-1.25)] = 1.25D. Stresspoint [4.00 + (-2.00)} = 2.00D. Bell [3.70 + (-1.70)] = 2.00D.

In patient A the difference in fixation distances are minimal [1"] and not clinically significant. We may reasonably conclude that all the measurements fall within expected levels of random measurement errors. Each of the four procedures has yielded similar diagnostic information.

In Patient B fixation distance varies from 16" to 10". To compare 10" and 16" observations requires converting these values to a common metric. This can be done graphically or by calculations described above. Also, these ratios may be referred to as slopes particularly when the retinoscope observations are graphed.

Patient A. The lag/distance ratios are: Book = 0.15, [.37/2.5]. MEM = .20, [.5/2.5]. Stresspoint = .20, [.5/2.5]. Bell = .14, [.33/2.33]. Differences in slopes equal to or less than .1 are not considered clinically significant. Discussion of the LN observations will be discussed with prescription criteria.

Patient B. The lag/distance ratios are: Book = 0.45, [1.12/2.5]. MEM = .50, [1.25/2.5]. Stresspoint = .50, [2/4]. Bell = .46, [1.7/3.7]. The similarities in lag ratios indicate that the same rate of change in accommodation has occurred as a function of changing target distance. Computed ratios allow easy comparisons from Bell data to MEM or vise versa. Theoretical predictions may be readily checked by direct observations.

Example: Suppose we wanted to predict an expected 10" MEM observation from the observed Stresspoint finding in Example B. Solution: Multiply Stresspoint lag ratio [.5] times the reciprocal of the fixation distance. Therefore, $_eMRL_a$ at 10" = [.5 x 1/.25cm] = -2.00D. This answer in diopters indicates that the estimated accommodative posture is 2 diopters behind the 25cm fixation plane and that the neutralizing sphere would be a +2.00D.

Conversions and predictions using gross targets as in these examples may be considered very probably within a range between 1m and 20cm provided the amplitude of accommodation is greater than 6D. This is true because accommodative behavior under binocular viewing with normal viewing conditions tends to be quite linear under dynamic retinoscopy with such targets and simple instructions. My infant studies[12] suggest that this linearity may extend over most of the accommodative amplitude range after 4 to 6 months of age.

Similarities and Differences in Lens Prescriptions

Similarities and differences in lens prescriptions resulting from these several retinoscopy procedures for the same task distance are dependent on many factors from random measurement errors to the specific or nonspecific prescription criteria used by the individual optometrist. Discussion is limited to listing previously reported prescription criteria and comparing these results with theoretical expecteds for Bell and Stresspoint findings and conversions.

For lens application, the primary diagnostic function which may be obtained from Book, MEM, Bell and Stresspoint retinoscopy is to determine whether accommodation is performing normally, hypo-posturing or hyper-posturing under various lens and task conditions. We assume that the observed responses to gross targets are representative of accommodative behavior under many normal environmental viewing conditions. The magnitude of the observed MRL_a under gross target conditions allows estimations of the corrective changes in accommodation required for fine discriminatory tasks such as stereo acuity, etc. Clinically, these objective procedures are attractive because they take little time to administer. Performance determinations, leading to a near lens prescription, may be made through the distance refraction, the habitual glasses, no glasses or any other examiner selected lenses. If desired, testing may be performed at the patient's preferred working distance. A nearpoint lens prescription can be developed without farpoint measurements with some of the procedures.

By starting with gross targets with simple instructions and tasks, a number of quantitative lens solutions become possible. It is easy to estimate and verify the magnitude of improved retinal image definition to each eye for a proposed prescription by optically reducing the motor response lag of accommodation to acceptable limits. Effective lens prescriptions can be designed to control unwanted disruptive corrective accommodative movements associated with either hypo or hyper-posturing.

These corrective accommodative movements are often generated by visual tasks requiring intermittent fine acuity and/or stereo discrimination, task determined changes in fixation distance, by abnormal motor hysteresis or by poorly sustained accommodative responses over time, among other reasons. Undesirable accommodative corrective movements can induce unwanted synergistic lateral vergence movements which require corrective movements. Both forms of corrective movements can result in many forms of poor coordination between accommodation and convergence.

In addition to the reasons above, the Combined MEM-LN technique was developed to have an easy clinical means of quantifying the probably magnitude of change in accommodation from spherical lenses which may modify convergence behavior through interaction. This capability allows reasonable clinical prediction of when and how much we can expect to alter phorias, fixation disparity, blur points and strabismic fixation, etc, with spherical lenses. An explanatory graph for plotting the Combined MEM-LN test result is displayed in Figure 1. Figures 3 and 4 display plots for hypothetical Patient A and B.

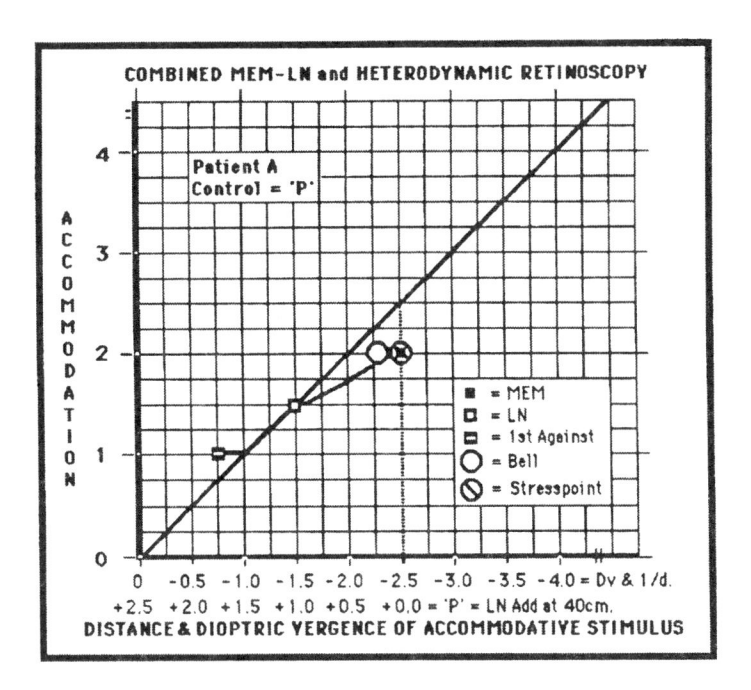

Figure 3. Patient A's Combined MEM-LN findings are plotted as a function of task distance and the plus sphere added to provide low neutral and first against observations. The initial MRL_a of -0.50 is reduced to 0.00D with +1.00D spheres [$ĆA_r$ = 0.50D]. Bell/Stresspoint are plotted as a function of 2D accommodative response and the reciprocal of distance in meters for eye to target distance. All findings indicate normal accommodative postural skills.

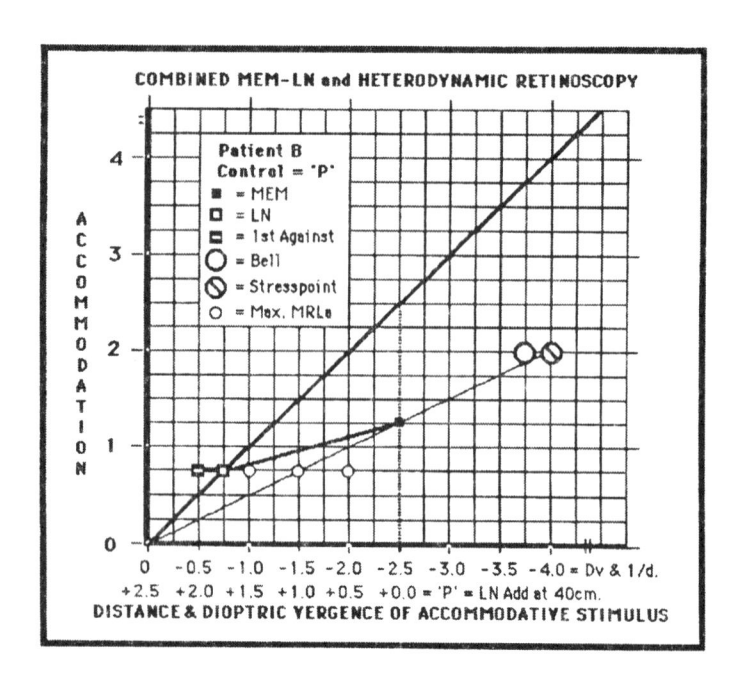

Figure 4. Patient "B" illustrates marked hypo-posturing accommodative disturbance on all tests. Linear increase in the MRL$_a$ is seen from 40cm to 25cm target to eye distance. Ratio of accommodative response to target distance is 0.5 for gross targets. Ratio of accommodative response to change in plus spheres when distance is held constant is 0.29 [.5 / 1.75]. Open circles equal maximum possible MRL$_a$ where accommodative response reduces to the LN level with introduction of first +0.50D spheres. Dark straight line between MEM and LN indicates gradual uniform reduction in accommodation to LN add [+1.75D]. Thin black line indicates expected Bell/Stresspoint finding on MEM slope.

Specific Quantitative Prescription Criteria

Below are listed specific prescription criteria for determining a nearpoint spherical lens prescription for each technique. Since Getman[13] has stated that Book retinoscopy was not developed for determining a near lens prescription and since the MEM and book are considered equivalent with suitable controls, only MEM criteria are described below. Similarities and differences are discussed following listing of the several criteria for each retinoscopy technique.

- **MEM**: While primarily designed as an isodynamic procedure to determine if lens intervention was indicated, several related prescription criteria have evolved.

    1. If a lens prescription for distance is indicated, then the MEM is administered through the distance prescription at about 40cm. If the observed motion is "with" and less than 0.75D, no different near lens is indicated. The MRLa is considered normal with the distance Rx. Image formation is adequate.
    2. If the observed "with" motion is greater than 0.75D then a nearpoint lens is indicated. Two prescription criteria have emerged. [a] The first criterion prescribes the full magnitude of the observed MEM. [b] The second procedure adds plus spheres binocularly over the distance prescription until the MEM motion attains a constant 0.50D "with" motion.
    3. If "neutral" or an "against" motion is observed, minus spheres are added binocularly until 0.50D to 0.75D "with" motion is seen. This becomes the recommended spherical lens prescription for both distance and near unless there are compelling reasons to the contrary.
    4. For infants and preschool children, the need for, and the magnitude of, a nearpoint prescription may be determined at near for hyperopes who have never worn a lens prescription. Distance refraction, while desirable, is not necessary and is recommended to be performed after the dynamic retinoscopy. MEM is performed without lenses at 40cm. If the observed "with" motion is greater than 0.75D, then a nearpoint lens is probably indicated. If anisometropia and astigmatism are observed, these are neutralized by appropriate lenses and the MEM procedure is carried out as described in #2 above. In many instances the magnitude of plus sphere by this criterion may be less than the magnitude of the hyperopia as measured by far. Also, see Combined MEM-LN below.

- **Bell/Stresspoint**: As I understand these hetero-dynamic procedures as advocated by Apell and Kraskin, the optometrist first chooses whether to administer the test through a distance refractive finding, a proposed lens prescription; or with no lenses when the patient has never worn glasses. With whichever choice, if "with" motion is seen when the bell is at the plane of the retinoscope [50cm] the bell is moved toward the patient until neutral or the stress point is observed. If the eye to bell distance is between 15" and 20" no additional sphere is indicated over the control condition. If the bell to eye distance is measured inside 15", plus is added in 0.50D steps, and the test is repeated until the bell is at the preferred distance range from 15" to 16". The magnitude of the sphere becomes the gross nearpoint prescription. In physiological terms, an excessive MRLa has been reduced to 0.50D to 0.62D at about 40cm while viewing the bell. [If "Against" motion is observed, the same procedure is used as was described in MEM-3 above.]

Theoretically, when the distance refraction is used as the control, this procedure will produce the same lens Rx as MEM-2b above. When no lenses are used as the control, this procedure corresponds with MEM-4 above. If Bell were administered with and without the distance refraction, there is good reason to assume the prescriptions would be similar in some cases and quite different in others. Such differences are explained by the different response patterns previously described by Haynes.[11] The Combined MEM-LN procedure was developed, among other reasons, to quantify and predict the differences in prescription values resulting from these different accommodative preset conditions. Absolute presbyopia is the limiting case where the magnitude of plus can be predicted with certainty by simple optical constructs.

- **Low Neutral [LN]** retinoscopy findings when used alone allow delineation of several additional prescription criteria.
  1. Low Neutral [LN] Normative method for 40cm gross lens value: Subtract LN population mean value from gross LN spherical measurement. Rx [LN] = LN gross + [-0.87D].
  2. Low Neutral [LN] practitioner desired MRLa at 40cm: Select desired MRLa when wearing lenses and subtract from LN gross. Suggested: Rx [LN] = LN gross + [-0.37D]. A similar procedure may be used for other task distances.

- **Combined MEM-LN**: Combining Low Neutral retinoscopy with the MEM procedure allows the direct clinical measurement of how the accommodative system responds to the change in the wavefront of the accommodative stimulus from lenses when distance, target, and instructions are held constant. Results of relative accommodative tracking are observed. Thus, we can reasonably measure how much a given sphere value will improve image definition and how much the lenses will change the accommodative response [physical accommodation]. Stimulus/response curves similar to those generated with various laboratory optometers may be obtained for clinical purposes. The following prescription criterion[14] for the Combined MEM-LN findings in a slightly different form was first presented to the profession at the 1987 COVD meeting in Philadelphia. This criterion includes the slope of the accommodative response ratio as derived from the initial MEM to the LN measurements. It was specifically designed for preschool and early grade school children to allow minimum plus lens prescription where either isodynamic or hetero-dynamic procedures indicate an excessive MRLa. The formula for the Combined MEM-LN Rx in gross form, when starting with no lenses, may be written as follows:

Rx [MEM-LN] = LN^d + [$_e MRL_a$ + (1 − (ΔA_r + LN^d))].
Where:

LN^d = Gross spherical value of lenses before the eyes when low neutral is seen.
d = Eye to retinoscope target distance in meters [40cm].

$_e MRL_a$ = Clinician desired MRL_a when patient wears near prescription. Use minus sign [-] followed by dioptrics value for desired $_e MRL_a$ [-0.25, -0.37, -0.50, etc.].

ΔA_r = Change in accommodative response obtained from MEM to LN, [ΔA_r = LN − MEM].

The above formula will provide the minimum plus sphere to obtain the practitioner desired MRLa. It assumes an approximate linear change in the accommodative response over the entire MEM to LN range. At LN level the MRLa = 0.00D. Figure 7 shows this outcome graphically by the black line from MEM to LN. The open circles on the graph indicates that accommodation is reduced equal to the dioptrics value of the lenses until the LN posture is achieved at which times the lenses simply focus the emergent light beam from the eye to the retinoscope aperture. This produces a maximum graphical solution.

A minimum graphical solution can be read by inspection by determining where the distance between the diagonal line and the MEM-LN line [min sphere] equals the desired MRLa value. The maximum plus required is determined by the distance between the open circles [Max MRLa] and the diagonal line which equals the desired MRLa value. This minimum/maximum solution is the reason the magnitude of motion is estimated while testing from MEM to LN measurement. This difference in accommodative response explains the fact that various magnitudes of plus spheres are required in two different cases where the retinoscope to target distance are the same with the Bell/Stresspoint techniques.

Three additional hypothetical examples C, D, and E are provided below to clarify the several prescription criteria and to elaborate on selected theoretically interesting concepts associated with lens prescriptions. Hypothetical Patient E shows calculation of various lens prescription values for near when the distance refraction is not used as a control or given. These last three examples are graphed in Figures 5, 6, and 7. For comparative purposes Table I tabulates the several independent prescription criterion described above for all five examples.

Examples: Patient C. Assume a 6-year-old 1.00D asymptomatic hyperope is examined where no lenses are used for the preset test conditions at 40cm with a 20/100 letter oral letter reading task. Results: Initial MEM observation = 0.25D "with" motion. Plus is added in 0.25D steps. First "neutral" [LN] is observed with +1.50D spheres. First observed "against" motion = +2.50D. See figure 5 for graph of findings. These results indicate an MRLa from plano to +1.25D spheres is equal to or less than -0.25D, from +1.50 to +2.25D = 0.00D ["Neutral"]; and +0.25D ["Against"] with +2.50D spheres. These results indicate that the accommodative response was maintained within 0 ± 0.25D over a range of 2.50D's lens change. This constitutes superior accommodative postural and relative accommodative skills found in approximately the upper 8% of children. Note that the accommodative response was made with a gross target. Therefore, angular size of the target is not a clinically significant control element of the accommodative stimulus. The child detected and responded to the incident wavefront of the dioptrics light vergence. With Bell retinoscopy, eye to bell distance would be expected at about 18". Since my infant studies[12] in 1962, I have had the hunch that these prescription criteria should be studied carefully as a possible aid to shaping normal refractive and accommodative development. It appears that Apell and Kraskin may share my hunch.

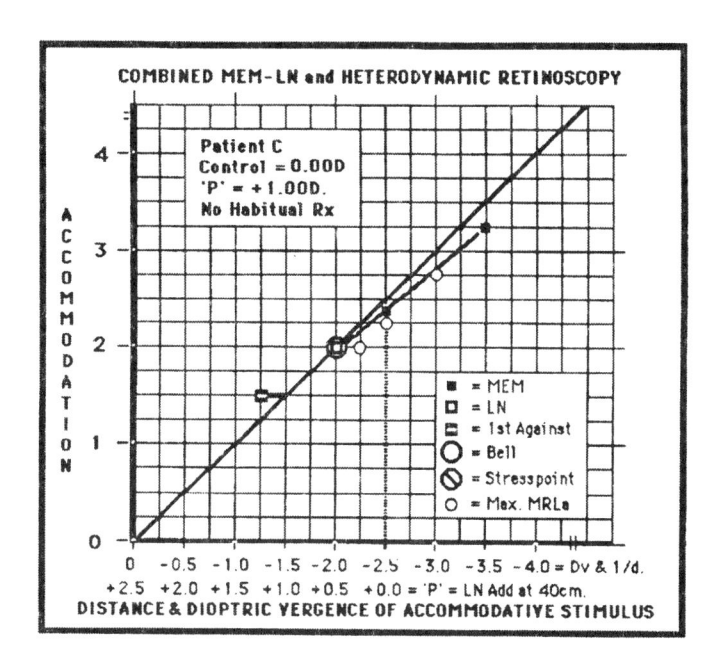

Figure 5. Patient "C" illustrates a 1.00D hyperope wearing no lenses during the initial testing with each retinoscopy procedure. All tests indicate normal to superior accommodative performance without any glasses. Ratio of accommodative response to change in target distance and to lenses from MEM to "first against" is 0.87D. The accommodative response is within +/- 0.25D of the fixation plane over a dioptric range of +2.25D.

Patient D. Assume a symptomatic child in terms of performance and asthenopia who is currently wearing a full distance hyperopic prescription. Control: habitual lenses. Findings: MEM = 1.00D "with" motion. Low Neutral = +1.00 add over habitual. First "against" = +1.25D.

Patient D's workup includes: MRLa with habitual Rx = -1.00D at 40cm. MRLa with +1.00 [LN] = 0.00D, A_L = +1.00 add. A_p = -1.00D from fixation plane. A_r = 1.50D at 16" with 20/100 letter reading. See Figure 6 for a graphical presentation. These results show that the accommodative response has not changed with the change in spheres. Any lens prescription up to +1.25D would not be expected to change any convergence tests because the accommodative response has not changed. Image definition in the proximal stimulus would be improved by lenses. Estimated Bell retinoscopy eye to bell distance = 30cm [11.8"]. Calculated from MEM lag/distance ratio = 0.4, and Response/distance ratio = 0.6.

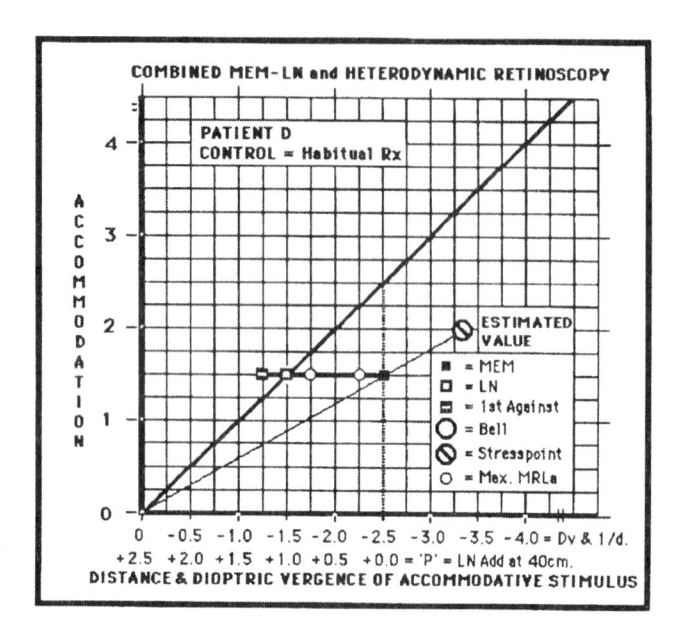

Figure 6. Patient "D" shows a rigid accommodative posture with a MRLa of -1.00D at 40cm through the habitual glasses. MEM equals LN. LN test lenses [+1.00] do not change accommodative response. Bell/Stresspoint is expected to be linear projection of MEM when accommodative response equals 2.00D [Eye to retinoscope = 50cm while eye to bell distance = 30cm].

Patient E. Assume a 4-year-old child in nursery school. No anisometropia or astigmatism. Findings are taken at 40cm. MEM = 1.00D "with" motion, LN = +2.75D, first against = +3.25D. MEM was taken with the Bird card with no discernable change in average "with" motion when the child is asked to tell the color of the eye or point to the eyes or other detailed features of the target. Figure 7 shows a graph of these findings. Since the distance refraction was not used as a control as in the previous examples all plotted data points constitute the accommodative posture relative to the target's 40cm fixation distance combined with the change in the dioptrics vergence as a function of the test lenses [plano to +3.25D OU].

MEM observations indicate accommodation is rigidly postured one diopter behind the fixation plane at 40cm. The magnitude of LN gross plus sphere and the magnitude of the change in accommodation from the test lenses suggest that the magnitude of hyperopia is probably between +1.50D to +2.00D. The change in the accommodative response is 1.75D, [LN + MRLa = +2.75 + (-1.00)]. The Combined MEM-LN near lens prescription to obtain an MRLa of -0.50D at 40cm is calculated as follows:

$$Rx\ [MEM-LN] = LN_d + [_eMRL_a + (1 - (\Delta A_r + LN_d))].$$
$$= +2.75 + [-0.50 + (1 - (1.75 + 2.75))]$$
$$= +2.75 + [-1.37] = \underline{+1.37D\ OU.}\quad Answer.$$
<u>Minimum Solution</u>.

This answer indicates that the least plus spheres to produce a "normal" MRLa [-0.50D] is substantially less than the estimated distance refraction [+1.75D] and slightly less than a diopters less plus than if the criterion [LN − 0.50D] were used. Theoretically, the Bell/Stresspoint procedures should provide a very similar lens prescription value if testing is started with no lenses.

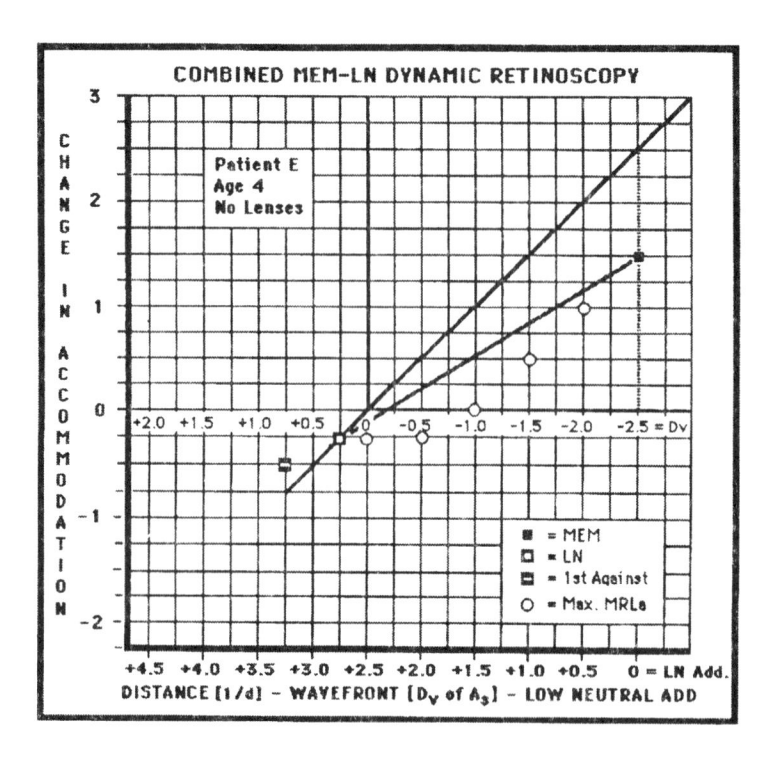

Figure 7. Patient "E" illustrates a preschool child tested without any lenses in the initial sequence. Distance refraction is not given. MEM at 40cm indicates a -1.00D MRLa which is not considered adequate during inspection of both gross and fine detailed objects for normal perceptual development. Retinoscope observations indicate partial sensory deprivation. Total change in accommodative response [ĊAr] to spheres [+2.75D] is 1.75D. See Table 1 for wide range of possible lens prescriptions depending on Rx criterion.

TABLE I. DIAGNOSTIC AND LENS PRESCRIPTION SUMMARY

CATEGORIES & Rx CRITERIA	EVALUATION OF LENS PRESCRIPTION CRITERIA				
PATIENT EXAMPLES	A	B	C	D	E
DISTANCE REFRACTION = ['P']	'P'	'P'	+1.00D	Habitual Rx	Not Given
CONTROL LENSES	'P'	'P'	NO LENSES	Habitual Rx	NO LENSES
40cm Rx Indicated: Book	NO	YES	NO	YES	YES
40cm Rx Indicated: MEM	NO	YES	NO	YES	YES
40cm Rx Indicated: Bell	NO	YES	NO	YES	YES
40cm Rx Indicated: Stresspoint	NO	YES	NO	YES	YES
40cm Rx Indicated: Comb. MEM-LN	NO	YES	NO	YES	YES
Gross MEM	No Add	+1.25 add	None	+1.00 add	+1.00D
MEM: Minimum Plus to -0.50 MRLa	No Add	+1.00 add	None	+0.50 add	+1.25D*
Estimated Bell/Stresspoint	No Add	+1.00 add	None	+0.50 add	+1.50D*
Normative: LN Gross + (-0.87) =	+0.12 add	+0.87 add	+0.62D	+0.12 add	+1.87D
LN MRLa: LN Gross + (-0.37) =	+0.62 add	+1.37 add	None	+0.62 add	+2.37D
Combined MEM-LN: Graph min. =	No Add	+1.00 add	None	+0.50 add	+1.37D
Combined MEM-LN: Graph max. =	+0.50 add	+1.25 add	None	+0.50 add	+2.25D

* Values assumes MEM-LN curve is linear. If curvilinear, and maximum MRLa, then the plus for -0.50D MRLa = +2.25D. See Figure 7 for the two curves defining Rx differences.

Table 1. Diagnosis of the need for a near point lens prescription by different dynamic retinoscope procedures and the several quantitative magnitudes of prescription values are summarized for each of the five example cases [A-E]. All five procedures are in agreement as to whether a near point prescription is indicated or not indicated. As seen above, the dioptric magnitude of prescription values may, depending on the case and the individual prescription criterion, converge of show wide variation.

Discussion and Summary

When appropriate mathematical models or graphical techniques are used for conversion of the different isodynamic and hetero-dynamic procedures using gross targets, all evidence indicates high agreement can be expected theoretically. Adequate empirical studies have not been performed to test this conclusion completely. All available clinical observations suggest similar conclusions. More agreement is evident as regards diagnosis of "normal" from "abnormal" accommodative performance than for the dioptrics magnitude of the near prescription. If reasonable optical controls are observed, each of these techniques should identify cases of hypo or hyper-postural accommodative disturbances as measured by an excessive MRLa. Clinical trials are indicated to determine how various prescription criteria may converge or differ, and to determine which prescription is most beneficial to the patient.

Only the Combined MEM-LN procedure is capable of quantifying relative accommodative tracking or supplying sufficient data to plot or calculate the slope of the MRLa. Estimating the actual change in the accommodative response as a function of a given nearpoint prescription for both gross and fine discriminatory tasks is best accomplished with the Combined MEM-LN. Reasonable results can be obtained from Bell/Stresspoint with gross targets by calculating the changes in eye to bell distance with each successive increase in plus spheres. This is a somewhat laborious task. None of the procedures used in isolation will identify those cases with normal postural accommodative performance and excessive ACA ratios leading to convergence in-coordination of various types, including strabismus.

Hypothetical Patients A, B, C, D, and E may be summarized as follows: All procedures would identify Patients A and C as having normal to superior accommodative performance which do not require a lens intervention as judged by observed accommodative performance with dynamic retinoscopy.

Patients B and D would be recognized by all as requiring a different lens prescription for sustained nearpoint tasks than for far. Hypo-posturing is present. Fine discriminatory targets and tasks would require excessive accommodative corrective movements. Symptoms are probable, depending on age, task complexity, duration and discriminatory requirements of the near visual tasks. These two hypothetical examples are illustrative of frequently seen clinical problems.

Patient E raises the important question of how much plus to prescribe for preschool children when the child's accommodative postural skills are not performing well. The prescription is written to allow the child to have "normal imagery" at near while at the same time providing a lens which allows reduction of infantile hyperopia without optical interferences with distance vision. Further, this criterion raises the often discussed question of what magnitude of the cycloplegic finding should be prescribed in a young hyperope? Certainly "full plus" is not indicated, unless adverse accommodative-convergence interactions are present and must be controlled as is the case of strabismus with a high accommodative component. The theoretical consequence of this prescription criterion needs careful investigation.

This very long answer to Dr. Flax's provocative question illustrates how much work has been done and how much is before us if we are to develop better knowledge about lens application procedures to shape, control and/or modify aberrant accommodative behavior.

References and Notes

1. Gesell A, Ilg FL, Bullis GE. Vision – Its Development in Infant and Child. Santa Ana, CA: Optometric Extension Program Foundation, 1998. Originally published by Harper and Row, Darien, CT, 1949.
2. Getman GN, Kephart NC. Book Retinoscopy. Santa Ana, CA: Optometric Extension Program Foundation Papers, 1958; Series 2 (10-11):65-74.
3. Haynes, HM. Clinical observations with dynamic retinoscopy. Optom Wkly 1960; 51:2243-6, 2306-9.
4. Apell RJ, Lowry R. Preschool Vision. St. Louis: American Optometric Association, 1959.
5. Apell RJ. Clinical application of bell retinoscopy. J Am Optom Assoc 1975;46:1023.
6. Streff, JW. Some Early Observations With a Bright Bell and Retinoscope. Eastern States VT Conference, 1962;36:416-9.
7. Kraskin RA. Lens Power in Action – Stresspoint Retinoscopy. Santa Ana, CA: Optometric Extension Program Foundation Papers 1982; 54 Series 1(7-8).
8. Sheard CA. Dynamic Skiametry. Chicago: 1920.
9. Sheard CA. A quantitative system of dynamic skiametry, Am J Optom 1929;6(12):669-93.
10. Haynes HM. clinical approaches to nearpoint lens power determination, Am J Opt Physiol Opt 1985;62(6):375-85.
11. Haynes HM, White BL, Held R. visual accommodation in human infants. Sci 1965;148:528-30.
12. Getman GN. Invitational Skeffington Symposium on Vision, January 1989, Washington DC. Dr. Getman during audience participation stated that he had never advocated Book retinoscopy for determining a specific nearpoint lens prescription value and requested that this fact be generally acknowledged. He indicated that Book retinoscopy was developed to gather developmental information particularly to study the effects of cognitive behavior on retinoscopy observations.
13. Haynes HM. Lecture supplement handout prepared for participating optometrists at COVD invited lecture. Philadelphia, PA, November 1978.

The Impact of Visual Training on Intelligence

Martin Kane, O.D., COVD
Philadelphia, PA

Abstract

Many of the most important skills that people possess are often overlooked in an optometric evaluation. These skills are the innate intellectual capabilities of the patient. Because they are not considered during testing, that is not included in the implementation of a visual training program. Confounding the problem is the notion held by psychologists that there exists but two types of intelligence – verbal intelligence and performance intelligence. In reality, there are a number of different types of intellectual potentials. These multiple intelligences include: linguistic intelligence, visual/spatial intelligence, logical/mathematical intelligence, bodily/kinesthetic intelligence, musical intelligence, intrapersonal intelligence and interpersonal intelligence. Each of these different types of intelligences has a significant impact on behavior. With an understanding of the various aspects of intelligence, optometric visual training activities can be designed and/or modified to enhance a patient's intellectual performance.

Introduction

Unfortunately, some of the most important skills that individuals possess are too frequently overlooked and totally ignored during visual training. These skills are the innate intellectual capabilities of the patient. Confounding this problem is the lack of understanding about the various types of intelligences. Most people concerned with human behavior, because of the nature and scope of intelligence testing, account for but two types of intelligence: the verbal skills (the ability to manage visually presented material). This overly simplistic approach to intellectual testing is extremely limited because it fails to investigate the complexity of intelligence and it neglects to consider those intelligences which are equally critical to effective behavior. These multiple intelligences are determinable, accessible, and trainable!

But just what is intelligence and how can it be defined? Let us start with two working definitions – one for intelligence and the other for visual intelligence. Intelligence is the skill or efficiency to internalize data, integrate it into an image (idea) and apply alternative strategies in using this image for solving new problems.

Visual intelligence is the skill or efficiency to internalize data, integrate it into a visual image and apply alternative strategies using this information for solving new problems. The word skill (Webster's Dictionary, 1972) implies that intelligence is an ability to use one's knowledge (past experiences and prior learning), effectively formulating ideas about how to execute a task. Also implied are the technical ability, proficiency and competence that a person can mobilize. To incorporate higher levels of intelligences, an individual creates ideas (images) about task resolution and applies a variety of different strategies to utilize these ideas to solve tasks that haven't been tackled previously.

Intelligence is dynamic and changeable. It is impacted upon by both the environment and by experience. The greater the amount of experience and exposure one has, the higher the intelligence. The converse is also true; limited experiences results in lower intelligence. Studies also indicate that verbal intelligence is extremely resistant to change and that performance intelligence is much more flexible. Research supports the conclusion that expectations and demands of society will increase or decrease one's intelligence.

Multiple Intelligences

There are at least seven different types of intelligence that can be identified. This list includes: linguistic intelligence, visual/spatial intelligence, logical/mathematical intelligence, bodily/kinesthetic intelligence, musical intelligence, intrapersonal intelligence and interpersonal intelligence (Gardner, 1983). Each of these potentials plays a different and significant role in the proficiency with which we manage information, interact with people, communicate ideas, solve problems and made decisions. After these intelligences are identified and understood, people can be shown how to access each of these potential skills. Then, training programs can be developed to enhance their effectiveness to meet both routine and complex demands. It is imperative to remember that no intellectual domain exists in isolation. All intelligences interact and impact on each other.

Linguistic Intelligence

Linguistic intelligence is the ability to understand and produce language, and to use language to solve problems. It allows us to access and understand our own inner language as well as the language of others. It provides us with the ability to think in language, create poetry, comprehend what we read, and understand written, spoken, and manual conversation. A high level of linguistic intelligence provides us with an opportunity to develop excellent command of language and, when we speak, to express ourselves effectively and succinctly. Hopefully, it prevents us from talking much while saying little.

A number of prolific writers come to mind when reflecting on those with a high level of linguistic skills. T. S. Eliot certainly exemplifies this skill. At the age of ten years, during a three-day period of time, Eliot wrote eight issues of the magazine he called "Fireside." Each issue consisted of poems, adventure stories, humorous items and a gossip column. He continued to write extensively and well for many years. Shakespeare, Dumas, Tennyson, Descartes, Kant and many others have demonstrated inordinate abilities in this domain.

Linguistic skills are critical in our daily activities. They provide us with the ability to listen and hear, to talk our way through a problem, to communicate with others by sending, receiving and understanding verbal and written ideas and directions, and more importantly, to "connect" with people. They allow us to establish goals, communicate our culture, and to deal with the day-to-day machinations of life.

Visual training can enhance linguistic intelligence if patients are required to explain what they are doing in each training task and if they are required to explain how they go about attempting to solve a problem.

Trainees should be taught to plan ahead, organize their thoughts and express their modus operandi. They should be provided with an opportunity to become the trainers in visual training and they should be required to find the language to explain to others what must be done to successfully complete a task.

Visual/Spatial Intelligence
Visual/Spatial intelligence is an ability to apply visual imagery to interpret, remember, reconstruct and understand our space world, and to remember that which we see. It provides us with the ability to produce in our minds-eye pictures of things we have previously experienced, and to remember and understand where and how things are located in space, to solve graphically represented puzzles or tasks and to create new visual ideas. Visual intelligence permits us to see the relationship amongst ideas and things, to create new tools and hardware, and to draw and paint pictures. And it allows us to rapidly draw conclusions. Remember, "A picture says a thousand words."

Leonardo Da Vinci was a visual genius, demonstrating marvelous skills in this type of intelligence. He sketched, painted, sculpted, and he created numerous musical and mechanical devices. The basketball player, Larry Bird, exemplifies high spatial skills. He was and still is always aware where the ball is going or needs to go, and where other players are located on the court. He is always in command of the action.

Visual/spatial skills provide us with the ability to profit from what we have seen before, to understand how things and ideas are interrelated and how things work, to see what is missing, to create new technologies, and to see (forecast) into the future. It is interesting to note that Confucius stated over two thousand years ago that we forget what we hear, but that we remember what we see!

Perceptual and cognitive training in conjunction with visual thinking and visual imagery, all routine techniques in visual training, impacts positively on intelligence. Other activities such as visual and spatial memory games, spatial localization tasks and puzzle manipulation also can be used to enhance this type of intelligence.

Logical/Mathematical Intelligence
Logical/mathematical intelligence provides us with the ability to apply and translate deductive reasoning into problems that can be solved via logic and/or mathematic computation. These skills give us the innate potential to systematically organize our thinking, to plan ahead, to evaluate critically, to develop alternative strategies to solve a problem, and to know when and how to take calculated risks. This type of intelligence provides us with the ability to understand mathematical

concepts and computations, and to understand the precise organization and spatial configurations, numbers and ideas.

No one can deny that Albert Einstein had to possess extremely high logical/mathematical intelligence in order to conceive of an idea as complex as the theory of relativity. Galileo, Newton, and Hemholtz certainly weren't slouches when it came to this type of intelligence.

Many of the skills important in routine problem-solving tasks are derived from our logical/mathematical intelligence. These include our ability to organize, plan ahead, analyze, synthesize and evaluate. The competency required in shopping for our needs and managing our money stems from this type of intelligence.

Perceptual and particularly, cognitive skill enhancement, when incorporated into a visual training program can, by nature of their construct, have a positive impact on intelligence. Critical to this type of training are task demands that require careful planning and organization, calculated problem solving, and the request to create alternative strategies when trying to solve problems.

Bodily-Kinesthetic Intelligence
Bodily-kinesthetic intelligence is the skilled control of bodily movements, and the ability to refine, continually, the movement of body parts to solve problems that require movement. This type of intelligence guides the efficiency and effectiveness of our hands, fingers, eyes, tongue, feel, and all of the other parts of our body when moving in space, or when interacting with objects located in space. It provides us with the ability to walk, run, swim and participate in sports and dance.

Julius Erving epitomizes this type of skill. When he was younger, he was capable of making movements in space that defied all concepts of the force of gravity. He was able to move his body proficiently into positions that were not previously demonstrated in basketball or any other sport. He revolutionized body movements of the game. A number of our highly skilled dancers, gymnasts and sports celebrities had very high bodily-kinesthetic intelligence. Rudolph Nuryev, Curt Thomas, Nadya Comenici and Babe Ruth come to mind.

Bodily-kinesthetic intelligence helps us to get into the rhythm and tempo of others, and into the flow of life. It provides is with many of the mechanical skills necessary to draw and write, and to operate typewriters, computers, machinery, tools and moving vehicles. It helps us to avoid many needless accidents. This type of intelligence is what accounts for the well-known adage: "we learn by doing." Confucius stated over 2000 years ago that "we learn what we do."

Visual training which includes gross motor activities (such as balance beam, balance board, trampoline, ball handling and any other task that required motor planning), and fine motor activities (such as visual tracking, and finger, hand and tongue control tasks) can enhance intelligence.

Musical Intelligence
Musical intelligence is the powerful and compelling reaction to sound. It provides us with the ability to appreciate, understand and reproduce sound/music. It accounts for our musical ear, and for our ability to sing and play musical instruments. It helps us to get into the swing of things!

Wolfgang Amadeus Mozart is an example of superior musical intelligence. At the age of four years, he was composing sophisticated music. Yehudi Menuhin, after hearing the violin for the first time at the age of three, demanded his parents get him one. He immediately sat down and played the instrument. Any number of highly skilled musicians can be named. Beethoven, Chopin, operatic composers, some of the members of the Beatles, Bacharach, Caruso, and Streisand are just a few.

Our musical intelligence also helps us to get in tune with people. It, too, helps us to follow the rhythm and tempo of others, and it helps us to get into the flow of action.

To enhance musical intelligence, visual training should incorporate metronome and rhythm activities, and sound discrimination, sound localization and sound/ground tasks.

Intrapersonal Intelligence
Intrapersonal intelligence is the knowledge of the internal aspects of self and the ability to access one's own feelings and emotions. It provides one with the capacity to effect changes amongst these emotions, to identify and label them, and to eventually draw upon them as a means of understanding and guiding one's own behavior. It allows

one to form a positive or negative self-image and self-worth. In short, it gets one in touch with oneself and it helps one to mobilize one's inner resources. It is this type of intelligence that helps me to understand and accept who I am, what I can do (and can't do), and what I must do.

People with high intrapersonal intelligence are comfortable with themselves and, as employees they are able to do what they have to do. They look to themselves for verification, truth and approbation. They mobilize their own resources and find motivation within themselves to do the best job they can.

Activities that require training patients to establish goals, to verbalize feelings and attitude about visual training and to express the changes they see occurring during training impact on intrapersonal intelligence.

Interpersonal Intelligence
Interpersonal intelligence is the capacity to notice distinctions among others – their moods, desires, motivations, temperaments and intentions and to adjust, adapt and blend harmoniously with people. Folks who possess a high degree of this type of intelligence emerge as corporate leaders.

Gorbachev, during his recent visit to the United States, certainly demonstrated effective interpersonal intelligence. He ingratiated himself with the media and with most of the people with whom he cam into contact. Martin Luther Kin Jr., Mahatma Gandhi, and, probably, John F. Kennedy were in the same league.

High interpersonal intelligence provides people with the ability to effectively communicate with and mobilize others, to know when to back off and how hard to push, and to encourage others to follow.

The interaction between patients and vision therapists, patients and doctors, and patients and parents supports enhancement of this type of intelligence.

Conclusions
Research indicates that intelligence is extremely dynamic, and that both experiences and the environment can be arranged to enhance intelligence. The intellectual capacity of people can be expanded when attention is given to skill, efficiency, imagery and alternative strategy

development, and to solving new problems in each of the seven different types of intelligences. Each of these multiple intelligences is accessible and trainable when the right kind of optometric visual training activities are presented.

Bibliography
Gardner H. Frames of Mind. New York:Basic Books, 1983.
Webster's Seventh new Collegiate Dictionary. Springfield, MA: G. & C., Merriam, 1972.

The Interplay Between Change and Restraint

Barry Millis, O.D.
Philadelphia, PA

Elliott Forrest wrote in, *Stress and Vision*,[1] "All life involves interplay between two factors: movement, action, or change on one hand, and apparent inaction, restraint, or resistance on the other." This complementarity of life is basic to an understanding of the relationships between heredity and learning as I have discovered from reading Gregory Bateson's, *Mind and Nature*.[2] My own ignorance of the genetics/learning relationship has been a weak spot in my use of the behavioral optometric model. I had been in the habit of talking comfortably to patients about stress-induced vision problems, but their questions about the influence of heredity caused me, at least internally, to squirm a bit.

There is a relationship between heredity and learning. As Bateson points out, all relationships are a product of double description. It is useful to think of the two parties or processes as two eyes, each with a monocular view, and together giving a binocular view in depth. This double view is the relationship.

Bateson emphasizes the importance of double or multiple descriptions as a basic aspect of mind. Sensory awareness depends on news of difference. Two points of view that are collected and/or coded differently result in extra "depth" metaphorically. The formal relations that occur between different events or things may be seen as a product of multiple descriptions. For example, comparative anatomy consists of the formal relations we perceive between creatures. My mind contains no creatures, only the ideas of them. Mind contains no material other than its own hardware – there are no frogs, rabbits, or eagles in my mind, yet from the multiple ideas of these creatures a variety of lateral extensions can be drawn. These relations, called abductions, between all forms or patterns are what makes science, art, religion, and even dreams possible. The anatomy and physiology of the body can be considered as one vast abductive system with its own internal coherence, and the environment in which the creature lives has its own internal coherence, although the two systems do not immediately share the ability to integrate. For any change to occur, a double requirement is imposed on the new thing. It must fit the organism's internal coherence and it must fit the external environmental requirements. Double description now becomes double specification.

Abduction occurs throughout successful vision training. The feeling of letting go through a minus lens to let the Marsden ball blur, must be transferred to the Vectogram with base-in disparity. The body awareness achieved at the chalkboard needs to be integrated into the use of pointers at the stereoscope. These learned abductions within and among the components of the visual system result in expanded depth within the mind. Of course, there is no "depth" or "space" in the mind, only a learned image of them based on a matching of internal and external coherence. For a creature to endure, change must occur in doubly defined ways. Generally, the body's internal requirements will be conservative. In contrast, a changing environment may require the organism to sacrifice conservatism. A good vision training environment makes the sacrifice as painless as possible.

This Interplay between change and restraint is powerfully expressed in the two stochastic systems of learning and evolution, a stochastic process is one that combines a random component with a selection process so that only certain outcomes are allowed to endure. Shooting arrows at a target results in a somewhat random pattern where the position of some arrows is preferred over others. Bateson considered evolutionary and somatic (learning and thought) changes to be fundamentally similar, although each is governed by rules of a different logical type. Logical type is best defined by example. A class of things is of a higher logical type than individual members of the class. A second example, the depth achieved by binocular vision is of a higher logical type than the Information from each eye individually.

Actually evolution and learning are each doubly stochastic. In evolution, there is an internal process where the shuffling of genes is random, with the matching of DNA molecules in reproduction serving as the selection filter. If the proposed change in one set of genes is too unusual, there will not be a viable embryo. The external process consists of an interaction between environmental pressures on the somatic structures and processes as the random element, and the genetic state serves as the selection device. Environment and physiology propose somatic change, and the current state of the organism as determined by genetics decides the viability. Interestingly, the first stochastic process is digital, while the second is analog. This dichotomy is the main reason, according to Bateson, that acquired traits cannot be directly passed on from one individual to its offspring. A quantitative or analog process cannot determine form. Space is quantitative – changes in the shape of space reveal form, but do not produce it.

Within the individual, the double stochastic processes of thought involve internal shuffling of ideas with the selections made by whatever forms of logic or rigor that the individual possesses. There is also the external presentation of random experiences that are filtered through whatever has already been learned and reinforced. It seems to me that the Right/Left modes discovered in split-brain research, represent the internal stochastic learning process. The Right mode functions as the random generator with the Left mode serving as the filter that allows some ideas to endure. If awareness of the Right mode is suppressed, the natural selection of ideas is made from a limited menu. Inhibition of the periphery is a blockage of the random, resulting in distortion of the stochastic process. When one's internal coherence becomes built upon excessive central concentration, and when this behavior is encouraged on a societal level, the global mind is skewed. A willingness to raid the random is necessary to be fully alive.

Let us back up and discuss adaptation, and how myopia could be related to the stochastic process of evolution. According to Bateson, there are hierarchical levels of somatic adjustment that range from particular superficial changes (most concrete) to deeper (more abstract) levels that involve more general adjustments with the most abstract level being total genetic control. In other words, somatic or genetic determination of a trait is not an either/or function – there is a relationship.

Superficial changes, serving as emergency measures, and not economical for long term use, lead to deeper more general adjustments called acclimation. In the early stages of the visual stress syndrome, the emergency measures are noted as disturbances within the accommodative/convergence system where a built-in buffer exists to absorb short term stresses. If the stress persists, a deeper adjustment becomes necessary, and acclimation occurs in the form of myopia, astigmatism, or binocular breakdown. Superficial flexibility is restored at the price of deeper rigidity.

It is apparent from watching myopes, that there is a level of learning to learn, i.e., many people seem to learn how to acclimate more quickly and easily. The runaway myopic progression, encouraged by the misuse of concave lenses, could accurately be called addiction. There is, however, a finite number of learning levels before the genetic limit is reached, where learning can no longer occur. To quote Bateson, "At what level of logical typing does genetic command act in the determining of this characteristic? The answer to this question will always take the form: At one logical level higher than the observed ability of the organism to achieve learning or bodily change by somatic process."

In my opinion, what is currently genetic is the option to become myopic. It is an option that has always been there for a significant segment of the population, but was rarely needed. The increasing occurrence of myopia as a somatic response to stress can have an effect on genetics at the population level. Remember, evolution is a doubly stochastic process. The external random process of environmental pressures on the somatic structures will produce those acclimations allowed by genetics within the individual. Change is proposed on the genetic level when enough Individuals exhibiting the favored change start matching genes. In pre-close work cultures the myopic option was spread throughout the gene pool. It now is becoming concentrated within the population specializing in academic achievement.

There appears to be a small population for whom myopia occurs early without any significant environmental pressures. It would not be unreasonable to suggest that this myopia is the result of mutation. Today's culture represents the first time in human history that congenital myopes can enter a gene pool that favors their mutation. Eventually the gene pool of the close work population will be heavily weighted with those who have the option to become myopic, and those who are myopic without choice.

Again remember, even congenital myopia does not mean the loss of all levels of learning. We may not be able to prevent the change in ocular structure, but there is still the question of how much myopia is genetic, and how much results-from addiction to concave lenses. Vision training is about learning to learn. We pull people outside of themselves to recognize the behavior that contributes to their vision problem, whatever it is. Out of that awareness comes a jump of logical type – the behavior that created the problem was but one of the choices they have.

The old behavior was a member of a class of behaviors that are possible, with some outcomes preferred over others.

References
1. Forrest E. Stress and Vision. Santa Ana, CA: Optometric Extension Program Foundation, 1988. ISBN: O-943599-00-8
2. Bateson G. Mind and Nature – A Necessary Unity. Bantam Books, 1979, ISBN: O-553-34575-3

The Baltimore Myopia Control Project-- A Major Turning Point For Optometry

G.N. Getman, O.D., D.O.S., Sc.D.
Waldorf, MD

This optometric event, which took place in the Fall of 1944, has so faded into the dim history of optometry that it has become somewhat of a mystery − a mystery only because there have been so few and incomplete references to it. How many of you have ever heard of the Baltimore Myopia Control Project? How many of you who have heard about it have a good idea on what it was, how it came about, who organized it, and what it produced? Of all the people intimately involved in this project, I believe I am the only optometrist still living who was actively involved in the analytical appraisal of the trainees − unless Dr. Sterret Titus − who would now be 93 years old is still living. Drs. George Crow, of Los Angeles; C. Vernard Lyons, of San Francisco; Henry Quick of Owego, New York; Sterret Titus, of Kansas City, Missouri; Sol Lesser, of Fort Wroth, Texas, and G.N. Getman, of Laverne, Minnesota, made up this part of the staff. George Crow was present for the first four weeks, and the rest of us each spent two weeks running analytical examinations on the trainees to check their progress, and to make recommendations on any needed changes in lenses and training programs.

The training program was administered under the direction of Ms. Arla Johnson (Mrs. George Crow) with the assistance of Drs. Violet Dorris of Denton, Texas, Anita Eberl of Milwaukee, Wisconsin, Mrs. Emily Bradley Lyons, of San Francisco, and Mrs. Betty Broadhurst of Los Angeles. These five very talented and deeply devoted women contributed service that was far above and beyond the call of duty.

Drs. E.B. Alexander and A.M. Skeffington, of the Optometric Extension Program, were directors of the project with the most valuable assistance of Dr. Ward Ewalt of Pittsburgh, who served as the liaison with the American Optometric Association under whose name the project was conducted. Dr. Ewalt was directly responsible for most of the preliminary arrangements required in the organization and implementation of this very involved and complex event. Dr. Mary Jane Skeffington, from St. Louis, Dr. Arnold Gesell and Moss Glenna Bullis, from the Original Yale Clinic of Child Development, were frequent observers of the project and made significant suggestions for its progress. Miss Bullis made pre- and post- developmental appraisals of all the trainees, and her report was a most significant addition to the final evaluation of the project.

This entire project came about as the result of a complete coincidence. Dr. A.M. Skeffington was enroute to the west coast back in early 1944, and while sitting in the train's club car, got into conversation with another passenger about what each did, and where each lived. The other passenger became interested in Skeffington's account of his wide travels in conducting seminars and congresses for optometrists. The other passenger was particularly interested in the information Skeffington gave him about myopia because his daughter was extremely nearsighted, and was receiving stronger prescriptions twice a year. Skeffington was asked if anything could be done for this girl and he immediately referred the family to Dr. George Crow, in Los Angeles for further evaluations and recommendations.

Optometric visual training was recommended and a two-month program was almost immediately started in Dr. Crow's office. The young lady made excellent progress and the parents were tremendously pleased with improvements in the visual performance they had never been told could occur. During this time, Dr. Crow found out these parents were the editors of *The Ladies Home Journal*. The ongoing conversations, and the parent's observations of what was going on in Dr. Crow's office brought more and more interest in what could be done for children by optometrists. Now, let's allow Dr. Crow, himself, tell this fascinating story.

From an original tape made for Dr. Arthur Hoare, Editor of the *Optometric World* in the mid 1960s.

Comments by Dr. George Crow on The Baltimore Myopia Control Project

> *I imagine from the correspondence that Alex has shown you that you know about the Gould's coming here and me working on an impossible myope of around 4 or 5*

diopters, and I have rather taken a licking than to take on the job in the first place. But, it was an assignment and we did it. As far as reducing myopia, that is a question. But the girl could see things she had not been able to see before without her lenses. The Goulds came out with her and I worked on Mrs. Gould because she had a real nearpoint problem. I do not remember now what she had in glasses but they were obsolete; didn't fit and apparently were years old. I don't recall. I have the record somewhere. Anyway, at the same time I was working on Cecily and Mrs. Gould, I had quite a few of the flyboys and Navy men. The Navy, and the Air corps sent me dozens and dozens for visual training. I imagine well over a hundred cases. We worked with over 225 or 250 from various branches of services. They were fine physical specimens; passed high in their mental and they were very desirable young men. Also some pilots that had taught flying in World War I, and these men were well along in their presbyopic years, but especially the Army Air Corps wanted them. We had a few of those. Mrs. Gould took her training and I fitted her with lenses along with Cecily taking her training and they had a chance to talk to these boys; heard the story about flunking their visuals. The Goulds were there for several weeks, and heard how the boys had gone for their tests and passed them, and the Goulds got very interested. They saw many of the other youngsters I was working on. The more they were around the more excited they got. When they went back home, Mrs. Gould had her first good reading glasses, and Mr. Gould said: "One thing that makes this whole Baltimore Project worthwhile, Mrs. Gould no longer has these stacks of manuscripts on her desk that no one can do anything with until she reads them. It has been a real traffic jam and now that desk is down to the size it used to be 15 or 20 years ago. I've got our money's worth of just that alone."

The project itself came up after the Goulds had gone home. It was cooked up after they got back to Baltimore. This first thing I knew there was this big deal on to show what we could do with myopes. I didn't want to have anything to do with it, but they always said: "You have got to come and help." so Arla and I did. I talked about it to an ophthalmologist friend of mine – he has a worldwide reputation and is a very fine person and one of the outstanding ophthalmologists and surgeons in the world, and a graduate, by the way, of Johns Hopkins. He said, "Well, George, this is only going to turn out one way. They have to bomb it – they have to sabotage it someway. You are walking into a trap." I asked him what I could do about it now that it has gone that far, and he said, "Well, you can't do anything. You might as well expect what is coming and do your damndest." I said, "That is what we are going to do."

So, it was September 6, 1944. There was going to be a three-month program of visual training back there. Ewalt was the go-between in setting this up. The Goulds rented some floors in a building that was arranged in training rooms and examining rooms, and the supply houses either loaned or rented the equipment for testing and visual training. There was a small reception room decorated with Gould's paintings. When I got there, there was a big excavation out in front of the building and they had put in extra power because of all the equipment we were bringing in. They went to a tremendous amount of expense. I have forgotten how many thousands of dollars it cost. The first thing I found out was that the original plan was that we were to select these cases that we wanted to work on. When I got there, Ewalt came in one day to tell me that the ground rules had been changed. Hopkins would choose the cases, test them and then send them over to us. I was all for turning around and going home but I could not very well do it with all this remodeling and equipping. It was just one of those things you could not walk away from. Anyway, Arla and I arrived and it was arranged that I was to be there a month, and Arla was to be there three months. At the end of two weeks, Sol Lesser was to come in to work with me for two weeks, and then he was to work for two weeks more than Hank Quick, or Sterrett Titus, or one of the other optometrists there. We had the best visual training staff in the country: Violet Doris, Anita Pearl, Emmy Lyons, and Miss Broadhurst from our office. There were a lot of people coming in and out. For instance, Jim and Beatrice Gregg from out here, Emmett Betts, Gesell, and flocks of people came in just to be observers. Glenna Bullis who was one of Gesell's top staff came to observe and test the kids. So, we went to work.

The morning came when we were all set up and in came the first batch of 10 or a dozen kids. As these kids came in, and as others came in, these were the worst looking kids I had ever seen in my life. They were myopes but they looked sick. They were undersized and some of the girls and boys were obvious endocrine myopes. Some of these youngsters were actually ill. Some of them only had a few teeth left, and what had not been pulled was decayed right down to the gums. Some of them I know had tuberculosis. The way they coughed! This was what they had picked out over at Hopkins and sent over for us to work with. So, we went to work. There weren't 10 out of the first hundred kids that I would have taken into my office without first sending them to a physician, a good endocrine man and a good dentist. They were terrible subjects to work on. The therapy staff pitched in and started in with the visual training. It was remarkable the amount of improvement we got on some of these kids. Some of them did not want to work but the staff got them to work. We certainly had been double-crossed, no doubt about it.

After I left, they found out down in Annapolis, through the grapevine, that we were doing some visual training on myopes. The Commandant down there contacted the project and talked the visual training staff into staying down late at night to take care of some of the midshipman from Annapolis that had flunked their visuals. Thirty-three men, midshipmen, some lieutenants, some of them were J.G.s. They came up two or three times a week at night after the project was closed around 8pm. They would do their visual training until about 11 o'clock then go back to Annapolis. Every one of those 33 passed their final visual with better that 20/20 acuity. Of course, this was a secret and no one at Annapolis, outside of the Commandant, knew it was going on and they kept it very quiet, so there was nothing official about it.

The final tests were made at the end of the project by Ward Ewalt and a couple of others but I did not go back to see the cases. There was only one very interesting thing that did happen when I left Baltimore. I went to Chicago and had to lay over there a night for change of train. The ophthalmological section of the AMA was meeting there. Roy Wetmore, President of Riggs, called me and said, "I want you to come over to my hotel. There are two or three men here I want you to talk to. They are very anxious to talk to you." He did not say what it was all about but I met him at his hotel. He took me down into a corner of the exhibit room where there were some men that knew all about what was going on down at Baltimore. They had some cases they had intentionally put into the project and they were watching these cases. They knew we had been double-crossed. I never inquired who they were but I knew they were ophthalmologists, some of them officials, officials of the section. Two of them were biased against any kind of visual training. Finally one of them left and there then just two of them were still there. They had tested some of the kids because they knew what was going on. They frankly admitted they had tested some of the kids. Finally one of them said to the man who was kind of on our side. "Well you know this can't succeed because if it did every textbook in ophthalmology would have to be rewritten. That is an impossible job. You tell me how to do that, and then we can consider some of the angles we cannot consider now."

A lot of things went on after we got back home. Final tests were run both at Hopkins and by our staff. The parents were enraged because the Hopkins staff yelled at the kids and got them so upset they didn't know what was going on. The parents were terribly upset, and I think the Goulds found out about it too. Some of the parents were delighted with our efforts. The kids were doing better in school, doing better work, and they had made gains the parents realized. The kids were dismissed with the understanding we would recheck them three months later. We found out that only four or five of the parents would take their kids back to Johns Hopkins because they would not have anything to do with them. Jerry Getman went back three months later and he and Glenna Bullis checked about 35 of the kids, and they had improved more after three months than they had when we finished with them. So it was really quite successful.

There was a lot of opposition, even from some of the classical optometrists and some of those at the optometry college level. But, there was a lot of improvement in those we were able to see again. Glenna Bullis, who was Gesell's right hand at the Yale Clinic, who knew more about vision than most people, saw things they had never seen at the Clinic and what happened at Baltimore changed the entire program at the Yale Clinic. Up until then they had viewed some of the Gesell films with Skeffington, who was then invited to stop off at the Clinic. Skeffington called their attention to many things in the film and this brought new interests on the part of Gesell and Ilg. Eventually, the whole program changed to a visually oriented program, as a result of the Baltimore Project.

Note added by GNG: The ultimate result of all this was the close cooperation between optometry and the Yale Clinic, and the milestone book: *Vision, It's Development in Infant And Child.*

As Dr. Crow has just commented, there were and are a multitude of stories that could be told about this project, it's participants, it's details, and all the events that could naturally be coincidental parts of such an elaborate event. We could spend a long time with these interesting stories. However, the really important aspect of all this is the influence it has had on the profession of optometry. These impacts can now be itemized as follows:

1. Of chronological importance was the introduction to Gesell and the Original Yale Clinic of Child Development in New Haven, Connecticut. As stated by Dr. Crow, what Dr. Gesell observed at this Baltimore Project changed the entire direction of all the research on young children in that Clinic. When Gesell invited me to be a part of the clinic program, he said, "We have pretty well closed the door on the development of infants into childhood. We realize now that the door still open is the one to the visual

development of the human child. This must not be left unexplored." This invitation, and the financial support arranged for the clinic by Drs. Alexander and Skeffington, opened the way for the four years of intensive study and observations of visual development in children, and the eventuating impact that brought a developmental philosophy into the routine practices of many behavioral optometrists. Now, 40 years later, optometry continues to provide clinical benefits to thousands of children---and adults---that no other clinical discipline has discovered or even begun to consider.

2. If the photos of this project were available to all, it would be apparent that every one of the trainees spent their training time <u>seated</u> at some instrument, or in some training procedure. Several of us who were intimately involved recognized that Dr. Henry Quick brought changes in concepts and routines that were in force, and these changes significantly influenced the trainee's visual performance and status. Dr. Quick insisted the routines be changed whenever possible to get patients up and moving around in their visual environment. Dr. Quick insisted that the structural restrictions of all the "magic" instruments being used, and the immobility of the individuals, were actually hindering the results and the progress being sought for each patient. From the Baltimore moment until this moment, in 1989, the developmental/behavioral optometrist has insisted that every VT patient have the most training time <u>outside</u> any constricting and restricting instrument – that the individual immediate exploration and application of the visual skills needed for the visual mastery of the lighted environment are of supreme importance. Further, an instrument that keeps the patient constricted and restricted to some sort of "black box" cannot under any circumstances, even vaguely surrogate for the visual exploration of the lighted environment. There is a time and place for the exploration and enhancement of certain visual functions that can only be approached in these instruments, which supposedly substitute for, imitate, and/or represent the visual space world in which the optometric patient must perform in daily life. However, the lessons learned at Baltimore have shown us why the contributions of Darrell Boyd Harmon have become so important to us in any consideration of how we reach for the routines needed in the training room. Many of us went to Baltimore with a belief that our VT successes were primarily due to the designs and operations of the instruments we

were using. Each of these devices had some inherent magic that was bringing the changes in the visual status and performance of our patients. All we needed was the right instrument for the specific symptom. This belief led every optometrist who provided VT for his patients to buy every newly touted instrument and device that came along. Each of these new instruments had some new gimmick that would "cure" some visual problem, and all we had to do to have success in VT was to obtain this instrument and find a place for it in the training room. This first realization came at Baltimore that *NO* instrument, of and by itself, would be the answer to any sort of visual problem. All any instrument can possibly do is to assist the optometrist in helping the patient to understand his visual problem, and to then show the patient how he can do something to bring changes in that visual problem. Baltimore brought us all to the realizations that *NO* instrument contains any specific magic. The magic is in the patient's understanding of his problem, and in his desire and motivation to do something about it. And probably even more important than all of this, Baltimore brought the early realizations that specific attacks on specific visual functions, such as "accommodative excess" or "convergence insufficiency," would not bring any persisting positive changes in a patient's visual status. Training had to consider the entire patient, not just the two end organs.

3. This comprehension of the limitations of every instrument we use brought us to a much more important understanding of the visual process and the individuality of each patient. Our clinical minds were now opened to:

   a. The importance of the patient's understanding of his visual problem;
   b. The patient's understanding of his responsibilities, that we can do absolutely nothing to him, changes will only be the result of what the patient does for himself;
   c. The importance of the breadth and the depth of the indoctrination we give to each patient, his family and his teachers;
   d. The magnitude of the motivations and the desire really present in each VT patient;
   e. The understanding we convey to the patient about the long range purposes and goals of the visual training program---that there is much more to all visual training

than a quick change in comfort and acuity, or the "need for glasses." The most spectacular difference between the young men from Annapolis, and the 111 youngsters chosen by John's Hopkins Department of Ophthalmology, gave us the insights that brought optometry out of "orthoptics" by the medical model and visual training on an optometric model. These 44 intervening years have brought daily proof that no instrument's targets contain even the slightest hint of the patient attitudes needed, no matter how stereoscopic, anaglyphic, polarized or electronic these targets may be, and this matter of patient attitude continues to be the major difference between the medical model and the behavioral optometric model.

4. At about this same Baltimore time (1944), a number of us were fortunate enough to be participants in the summer courses being held in the experimental psychology department of Ohio State University with Professor Samuel Renshaw. Here we were exposed to notions and concepts about vision and visual performance in the human that challenged us to look carefully at the results of the Baltimore Project---and at the changes we expected which did not occur. Renshaw, and the Skeffington translations of the work, brought us quantum leaps away from the old ideas regarding the clarity of retinal images, and the classically exaggerated importance of the fovea and the central retina. As these new concepts were added to our moves out of the restricting instruments, into the emphasis being given to training procedures involving the patient in the open environment, we obtained new understandings and appreciations of what the peripheral retina was for, and how it could be stimulated to the patient's benefit. Dr. Sol Lesser, of Fort Worth, Texas, had already brought some rather special instrumentation to the Baltimore Project, but in mid-1945 he bought some sheets of Polaroid materials to Ohio State that had been carefully smuggled out of an experimental center by one of his patients. Dr. Lesser had already done some experimenting with polarized targets and Polaroid lenses worn by the patient. He found patients could experience widely ranging changes in the spatial orientations to items being so viewed when the retinal periphery was the primary area being stimulated while central retina viewing was held on unchanging central targets. All of this very emphatically brought new recognitions of why some of the

Baltimore patients made progress, which others did not make. The move out of the instruments, and the greater participations of the body as the reinforcing supporting structure for vision, brought significant advancements in the visual performance of some patients. We now achieved new appreciations of the role the peripheral retina could play in the patient's interpretations of visual space. Baltimore and Ohio State were tremendously serendipitous experiences that opened whole new clinical vistas to us.

5. Although Skeffington had been emphasizing the importance of plus lenses for all near-centered visual tasks since the early 1930s for all B1, and B2 type cases, and for all myopes, many of us failed to understand some of the reasons for plus lenses when the patient could see clearly without them. We easily appreciated Skeffington's insistence that plus lenses could be used for "esophores" because we could so frequently make immediate measurements of phoria changes brought by the plus. In Skeffington's February 1938 chapter (OEP Curriculum), he especially emphasized the use of plus on the myope to bring "greater coordination of functions which are referred to when we speak of the visual reflex, or the learned associations between accommodation and convergence." Again, in December 1942, Skeffington wrote about the importance of the plus lenses that should be used along with the visual training program for the myope. In spite of all of Skeffington's insistence and repeated emphasis, there was too much general consensus that it was really the visual training that brought the results--- not these plus lenses the patient did not need for clarity at near distances. Everyone was quite agreeable that myopes would probably do better with plus at near that "neutralized" the minus power prescribed for far, but there still was not the full appreciation of why there should be the stabilizing and enhancing plus lenses for all near tasks in which the myope was involved. It was the Baltimore Project and the concurrent explorations at Ohio State that impacted upon us. The probes of what changes in spatial discriminations and judgments the patient could appreciate through plus lenses brought great changes in optometric thinking in the late 1940s. Realizing that the usual myope has apparently lost sensitivity to visual periphery (as so frequently demonstrated by Dr. Sol Lesser's Polaroid ring routines), and that the introduction of plus lenses can also heighten peripheral awareness (also vividly demonstrated by responses to

Lesser's Polaroid ring routines), brought added attention to the importance of plus lenses for much more than the influences upon the "learned association between accommodation and convergence." Again, Baltimore and Ohio State in combination raised behavioral optometry to new levels of clinical abilities.

6. There is only one more aspect of this entire Baltimore Project that must not be overlooked. Many optometrists, who found themselves deeply involved in the visual training to enhance the acuities of young men and women striving for 20/20, demanded by some of the armed services, were very aware of changes in much more than acuity. Since optometry was so diligently trying to become a distinct clinical discipline, many optometrists were just as diligently avoiding any speech or behavior that might lead others to think these clinicians were imitating, or pretending to be psychologists--- or some sort of psychotherapist. Thus, many of the changes in the patient's social and interpretational behavior were either never mentioned, or if they were, it was only discussed in the deepest privacy of small bull sessions. Because of Miss Glenna Bullis' acumen in observing and reporting human development and behavior, she was invited to interview and survey the Baltimore trainees at the beginning of the project, at the end of the three months, and again five months after the project was completed. Her final report contains such comment as: "...their adjustment to the situation (in new surroundings and to the unfamiliar interviewer) was in marked contrast to their first visit in September. They looked more mature (more than five months gain), showed no shyness in approach, or in response to the questioning. <u>School</u>: A large percentage of the children reported improved school grades...even where marks had not been actually raised the children were finding "work" easier for them. <u>Sports</u>: Abilities in sports showed improvements comparable to that in scholastic gains...Two who were poor before made the baseball team...(others) were now enjoying active play. <u>Personality changes</u>: The obvious change in general demeanor has already been noted. Due to more facility with concentrated work and new participation in sports, the children's' lives have become fuller and more balanced." This report was written in mid-1945 for publication in January, 1946.

Ewalt, in his report to the AOA, wrote: "From the viewpoint of an adequate visual health care program for children, these changes are even more important than the improved vision. Such changes usually result from optometric visual training and are not limited to the training of near-sighted patients." Here for the first time, there was a public statement of the <u>total</u> changes in patients' self-esteem and their improved abilities to cope with the world and its challenges. This was still another of the differences the optometrist should recognize when comparing the camera model of ocular functions and the optometric model of visually influenced human behaviors.

As previously noted, a discussion of the Baltimore Myopia Project could go on and on because of the changes it brought in thinking and practices of many optometrists. These six points have been offered here as a brief account of why I personally think this project was a *MAJOR TURNING POINT FOR OPTOMETRY*. From my personal bias in human development, and my deep interest in children's early years, I have frequently referred to the Baltimore Project as the event that moved optometry from <u>infancy</u> to <u>childhood</u>. It moved us from the restrictions and confinements of the infant's crib structured on the classical philosophies by the camera model---to the open spaces of the new knowledge and abilities found by the child now confident enough of himself to cast off and search the new challenges being offered by the optometric model of the total person in whom vision is the dominant factor in all human behavior.

This turning point, from infancy into childhood, came to optometry because the Baltimore Project happened. Of course, it has been condemned, criticized and denigrated extensively by the non-optometric discipline, probably for the very reasons Dr. Crow reported after his stop-off in Chicago. Some of the criticisms brought by non-optometrists, and even some optometrists, are difficult to understand because they so clearly show such a paucity of understanding of the role that vision plays in all human performance. However, there are some reevaluations being made of the clinical data gathered at Baltimore, and these vividly reveal another myopia, myopia that no plus lens power will ever affect, and a myopic condition that no amount of training will ever change. Out of all this comes the really important realization that here was first major verification that optometry is a unique profession, one that never needs to fall back on imitation or parroting of some less informed group to build a façade of either self confidence or clinical status. This Baltimore Project should be a required course of study for <u>every</u> optometrist at <u>every</u> level--student, new graduate, short time practitioner, and the senior colleague. It must not be lost in the mysteries of dimming optometric history.